# Study Guide to Accompany Clinical Drug Therapy

## RATIONALES FOR NURSING PRACTICE

**Fourth Edition**

**GAIL ROPELEWSKI-RYAN,** RN, BSN, MSN

PROFESSOR

NURSE EDUCATION, HEALTH, PHYSICAL EDUCATION AND RECREATION

CORNING COMMUNITY COLLEGE

CORNING, NEW YORK

**ANNE COLLINS ABRAMS,** RN, MSN

ASSOCIATE PROFESSOR

DEPARTMENT OF BACCALAUREATE NURSING

COLLEGE OF ALLIED HEALTH AND NURSING

EASTERN KENTUCKY UNIVERSITY

RICHMOND, KENTUCKY

**J.B. Lippincott Company**
Philadelphia

Sponsoring Editor: Margaret Belcher
Coordinating Editorial Assistant: Emily Cotlier
Production Manager: Janet Greenwood
Production/Composition: Berliner, Inc.
Printer/Binder: Courier/Kendallville
Cover Printer: New England Book Components

Fourth Edition

6 5 4 3 2 1

ISBN 0-397-55184-3

⊛ This Paper Meets the Requirements of ANSI/NISO 239.48-1992 (Permanence of Paper).

*To my husband John,
my children Christine and Paul,
and to Carole and Julie, for their invaluable help and support.*

# Introduction

The *Study Guide to Accompany Clinical Drug Therapy: Rationales for Nursing Practice,* fourth edition, has been developed to complement Anne Abrams' text. It provides a wealth of learning opportunities to reinforce content that students have read in the text and to promote their ability to apply this information in the patient care setting.

Pharmacology is a tough and demanding science, fraught with seemingly limitless detail about an ever-growing number of drugs. Helping students learn the principles of pharmacology as applied to nursing practice to foster safe and effective management of drug therapy is perhaps one of the most challenging tasks surrounding nursing education today.

The *Study Guide* offers a variety of activities that incorporate approaches to learning designed to accommodate many student learning styles and increase the appeal of learning. The exercises have been chosen to help students establish a connection between how a drug works and why it is used for a particular disorder.

The *Study Guide* will help prepare students in the following ways:

- *Prepare for NCLEX test-taking:*
  NCLEX-style multiple-choice questions in every chapter give students an opportunity to practice their test-taking skills.

- *Develop critical thinking skills:*
  Case study exercises challenge students to develop their critical thinking skills and help students explore how they would apply those skills in a clinical situation.

- *Develop insight about client teaching needs:*
  Each exercise is aimed at expanding the students' knowledge base and understanding of drug therapy and increasing students' understanding of what patients need to know to maximize their drug therapy. Students will use information from the text to develop a teaching plan for persons who will require medication when they return home.

- *Receive immediate reinforcement of learning:*
  Answers for the multiple-choice questions and exercises are provided in the back of the workbook, allowing immediate feedback about the correctness of exercise answers.

- *Expand personal understanding of drug therapy:*
  Completing the exercises and working through the case studies provides valuable opportunity for students to immediately enhance learning effectiveness, building on classroom lectures, textbook reading and reflection, and completion of exercises provided at the end of each text chapter.

# Contents

# SECTION V. NUTRIENTS, FLUIDS, AND ELECTROLYTES

# SECTION VI. DRUGS USED TO TREAT INFECTIONS

# SECTION VII. DRUGS AFFECTING THE IMMUNE SYSTEM

# SECTION VIII. DRUGS AFFECTING THE RESPIRATORY SYSTEM

# SECTION IX. DRUGS AFFECTING THE CARDIOVASCULAR SYSTEM

# SECTION X. DRUGS AFFECTING THE DIGESTIVE SYSTEM

## SECTION XI. DRUGS USED IN SPECIAL CONDITIONS

# Study Guide
# to Accompany
# Clinical Drug Therapy
## RATIONALES FOR NURSING PRACTICE

**Fourth Edition**

# SECTION I

## Introduction to Drug Therapy

---

### CHAPTER 1

### Introduction to Pharmacology

---

## Matching exercise: terms and concepts

_____ 1. The study of drugs.

_____ 2. An individual drug that represents a group of drugs.

_____ 3. Chemicals that change functions of living organisms.

_____ 4. A group of drugs with common characteristics or uses.

_____ 5. The law that regulates distribution of narcotics and other drugs of abuse.

_____ 6. A process by which oral drugs commonly move from the GI tract to the bloodstream and from the bloodstream to cells.

_____ 7. A term used to describe processes a drug goes through after it enters the body.

_____ 8. Process by which a drug enters the bloodstream.

_____ 9. Process by which a drug is eliminated from the body.

_____ 10. Drugs stimulate liver cells to produce large amounts of drug-metabolizing enzymes.

_____ 11. Time required for serum concentration of a drug to decrease by 50%.

_____ 12. A substance taken by pregnant women that causes birth defects in infants.

_____ 13. When one drug removes another drug from binding sites on plasma proteins.

_____ 14. An adverse effect involving the liver.

_____ 15. An allergic response to a drug.

A. Drugs.

B. Controlled Substances Act.

C. Enzyme induction.

D. Pharmacology.

E. Prototype.

F. Absorption.

G. Drug classification.

H. Excretion.

I. Distribution.

J. Serum half-life.

K. Diffusion.

L. Displacement.

M. Hepatotoxicity.

N. Hypersensitivity.

O. Teratogen.

## True or false

_____ 1. Drugs are obtained from plant, animal, and mineral sources as well as being made synthetically.

_____ 2. Drugs in Schedule I have been approved for medical use and have no potential for abuse.

_____ 3. Routes of administration affect drug actions and responses largely by influencing absorption and distribution.

_____ 4. The action of a particular drug may be increased or decreased by its interaction with another drug in the body.

_____ 5. The effects of age on drug action are most pronounced in young adults.

_____ 6. Psychologic considerations influence individual responses to drug administration, although specific mechanisms are not known.

_____ 7. Drug dependence may be physiological or psychological.

_____ 8. Drug tolerance is a situation in which the body becomes accustomed to a particular drug over time so that larger doses must be given to produce the same effects.

_____ 9. Adverse effects are always life-threatening.

_____ 10. In elderly adults, physiologic changes may alter all pharmacokinetic processes.

_____ 11. Most oral drugs are excreted in bile, then eliminated from the body in feces.

_____ 12. Many drugs do not enter the brain and CSF, at least in therapeutic concentrations, because they cannot pass the blood-brain barrier.

_____ 13. Drug molecules bound to plasma proteins are pharmacologically active.

_____ 14. Drug movement and, therefore, drug action are affected by a drug's ability to cross cell membranes.

_____ 15. Pharmacokinetics includes the four processes a drug undergoes after entering the body: absorption, distribution, metabolism, and excretion.

## Cell physiology exercise

**Part A.** Fill in the blanks in Figure 1-1 with the terms below:

Golgi apparatus
Cytoplasm
Endoplasmic reticulum
Nucleus
Ribosomes

Cell membrane
Mitochondria
Chromatin
Lysosomes

**Part B.** Explain the relationship between the physiology of a body cell and the pharmacodynamics of a drug.

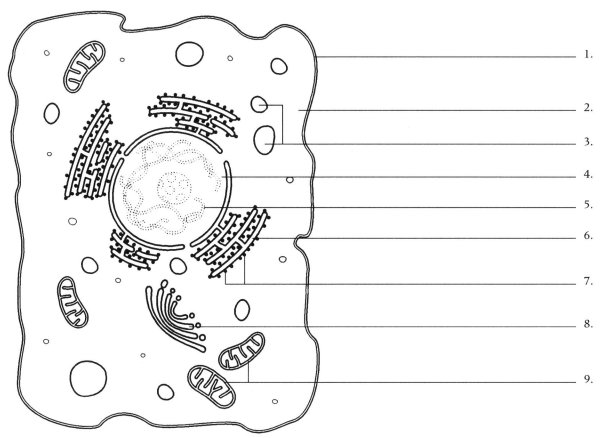

1.

2.

3.

4.

5.

6.

7.

8.

9.

**Figure 1-1**

## Review questions

1. The designated name given to the drug by the manufacturer who holds the patent:
   a. Generic name.
   b. Chemical name.
   c. Trade name.
   d. Family name.

2. You are caring for a client with cancer who has a low serum albumin. This concerns you because
   a. this will decrease the free drug available and reduce its effect.
   b. decreased albumin level decreases absorption.
   c. the client will have difficulty metabolizing drugs.
   d. most medications are bound to albumin.

3. Which of the following factors has the most significant effect on a client's response to medication?
   a. Sex.
   b. Climate.
   c. Age.
   d. Time of administration.

4. Half-life
   a. is a determining factor for how medication is administered.
   b. is decreased in persons with renal disease.
   c. may be increased if you double the dose.
   d. is not affected by the route of administration.

5. You have finished your teaching with Mrs. H. about erythromycin. You know that Mrs. H. has understood your teaching if she states that taking erythromycin with food will

   a. increase the rate of absorption.
   b. slow the rate of absorption.

   c. have no effect on absorption.
   d. significantly decrease the amount of drug absorbed.

6. You instruct your client not to take milk with tetracycline because

   a. an increase in stomach pH will decrease absorption.
   b. protein decreases metabolism of certain drugs.

   c. calcium binds with tetracycline and decreases its absorption.
   d. protein decreases absorption in the stomach.

7. An unexpected reaction to a drug the first time it is given is:

   a. idiosyncratic response.
   b. cross tolerance.

   c. hypersensitivity.
   d. hepatotoxicity.

8. Mr. J., a 65-year-old man with a long history of alcoholism, requires large amounts of pain medication following surgery. This may be due to

   a. idiosyncratic response.
   b. cross tolerance.

   c. hypersensitivity.
   d. hepatotoxicity.

9. The concurrent use of MAO inhibitors and food containing tyramine can cause

   a. fatigue.
   b. hyperglycemia.

   c. hypertension.
   d. respiratory distress.

10. When two drugs are administered together and the result is a decrease in the action of one or both of the drugs, this is referred to as

    a. synergism.
    b. displacement.

    c. antagonism.
    d. interference.

# CHAPTER 2

# Administering Medications

## Matching exercise: terms and concepts

_____ 1. One acceptable site for IM injections.

_____ 2. Both eyes.

_____ 3. Narcotic analgesics and other drugs with potential for abuse.

_____ 4. One ounce.

_____ 5. Before meals.

_____ 6. Units of measurement in the metric system.

_____ 7. IV, IM, SC injections.

_____ 8. Glass containers that may contain one or several doses.

_____ 9. An acceptable site for SC injections.

_____ 10. Under the tongue.

_____ 11. Glass containers that contain approximately one dose of a drug.

_____ 12. An anatomical landmark for administering an injection in the dorsogluteal area.

_____ 13. An anatomical landmark for administering an injection in the deltoid muscle.

_____ 14. A drug preparation suitable for use in the eye.

_____ 15. A dosage form designed to dissolve in the small intestine rather than in the stomach.

A. Controlled drugs.

B. Ventrogluteal area.

C. 30 ml.

D. a.c.

E. Meter, gram, liter.

F. OU.

G. Parenteral.

H. Vials.

I. Abdomen.

J. Sublingual.

K. Dermatologic.

L. Ampules.

M. Acromion process.

N. Ophthalmic solution.

O. Greater trochanter of femur.

P. Enteric coated.

Q. 240 ml.

## Abbreviations and equivalents

Match the definition in the right column with the abbreviation in the left column. Each definition can be used only once.

### PART I. ABBREVIATIONS

_____ 1. q.d.                 A. Right eye.

_____ 2. p.r.n.               B. Intramuscular.

_____ 3. q.i.d.               C. Immediately.

_____ 4. stat.                D. Sublingual.

_____ 5. q.h.                 E. Left eye.

_____ 6. h.s.                 F. When needed.

_____ 7. IM.                  G. Four times daily.

_____ 8. SL.                  H. Oral.

_____ 9. PO.                  I. Once daily.

_____ 10. OD.                 J. Every hour.

                              K. Bedtime

### PART II. EQUIVALENTS

_____ 1. 0.6 g.               A. 0.3 g.

_____ 2. 60, 64, or 65 mg.    B. 30 cc.

_____ 3. 1000 ml.             C. 1 gr.

_____ 4. 8 oz.                D. 10 gr.

_____ 5. 300 mg.              E. 600 mg.

_____ 6. 650 mg.              F. 1 tsp.

_____ 7. 30 ml.               G. 1 kg.

_____ 8. 5 ml.                H. 1 liter.

_____ 9. 2.2 lb.              I. 1 lb.

_____ 10. 1 liter.            J. 1 tbsp.

                              K. 250 ml.

                              L. 1 quart.

## Dosage calculations

### PRACTICE SET I

Determine how much medication you will administer:

1. Order: Ferrous sulfate 300 mg PO          Label: Ferrous sulfate 325 mg/tablet

2. Order: Penicillin 500,000 units IV          Label: Penicillin 20 million units in 20 ml

3.  Order: KCl 20 mEq PO                    Label: KCl 10 mEq/15 ml

4.  Order: Digoxin 0.25 mg PO               Label: Digoxin 0.125 mg/tablet

5.  Order: Atropine 0.6 mg IM               Label: Atropine 0.4 mg/cc

6.  Order: Demerol 30 mg IM                 Label: Demerol 50 mg/cc

7.  Order: Gentamicin 65 mg IV              Label: Gentamicin 80 mg/2 ml

8.  Order: Aminophylline 0.5 g IV           Label: Aminophylline 500 mg/10 cc

9.  Order: Heparin 3000 units IV            Label: Heparin 1000 units/ml

10. Order: Digoxin 0.25 mg IM               Label: Digoxin 0.5 mg/2 cc

11. Order: Cefadyl 500 mg IV                Label: Cefadyl 1 g/10 cc

12. Order: Valium 7.5 mg IM                 Label: Valium 10 mg/2 ml

## PRACTICE SET II

1.  Two ounces are equivalent to how many ml?

2.  The physician writes an order for 1 gm of aspirin. Each tablet contains 5 grains. How many tablets will you administer?

3.  Mr. J. is to receive 12 ounces of magnesium citrate. How many milliliters should he receive?

4.  Mr. P. weighs 132 lbs. How many kilograms does he weigh?

5.  You want Mrs. S. to drink 1.25 liters of solution. How many milliliters is she expected to drink?

6.  The physician writes an order for 125 mg. The bottle is marked 50 mg per ml. How many milliliters will you administer?

7.  The order reads: administer 20 grains. On hand you have grams. How many grams will you administer?

8. An ampule contains 50 mg of a drug in 2 ml of solution. The physician orders 10 mg of the drug. How many milliliters will you administer?

9. The order reads: administer 2500 units of heparin SC. The vial contains 10,000 units/ml. How many milliliters will you administer?

10. The order reads: give 10 ml of a solution. Mrs. J. wants to know how many teaspoons or tablespoons this equals. What would the best answer be?

## Review questions

1. Order: Aspirin 10 gr. PO.
   Label: Aspirin 325 mg/tablet.
   Administer:

   a. 1 tablet.  
   b. 1½ tablet.

   c. 2 tablets.  
   d. 2½ tablets.

2. Order: Penicillin 1,000,000 units IV.
   Label: Penicillin 20 million units in 20 ml.
   Administer:

   a. 0.5 ml.  
   b. 1 ml.

   c. 1.5 ml.  
   d. 2 ml.

3. Order: KCl 30 mEq PO.
   Label: KCl 10 mEq/10 ml.
   Administer:

   a. 10 ml.  
   b. 15 ml.

   c. 20 ml.  
   d. 30 ml.

4. Order: Digoxin 0.375 mg PO.
   Label: Digoxin 0.125 mg/tablet.
   Administer:

   a. 1 tablet.  
   b. 3 tablets.

   c. 4 tablets.  
   d. 5 tablets.

5. Order: Atropine 0.2 mg IM.
   Label: Atropine 0.4 mg/cc.
   Administer:

   a. 0.75 cc.  
   b. 1.25 cc.

   c. 0.50 cc.  
   d. 1.75 cc.

6. Order: Demerol 20 mg IM.
   Label: Demerol 50 mg/cc.
   Administer:

   a. 0.4 cc.  
   b. 0.5 cc.

   c. 0.6 cc.  
   d. 0.75 cc.

7.  Order: Heparin 7500 units SC.
    Label: Heparin 10,000 units/ml.
    Administer:

    a.  0.25 ml.                    c.  0.75 ml.
    b.  0.5 ml.                     d.  1 ml.

8.  Order: Gentamicin 60 mg IV.
    Label: Gentamicin 80 mg/2 ml.
    Administer:

    a.  1.582 ml.                   c.  1.384 ml.
    b.  1.500 ml.                   d.  1.486 ml.

9.  Order: Aminophylline 0.75 g IV.
    Label: Aminophylline 500 mg/10 cc.
    Administer:

    a.  1 cc.                       c.  150 cc.
    b.  15 cc.                      d.  1000 cc.

10. Order: Heparin 4000 units IV.
    Label: Heparin 1000 units/ml.
    Administer:

    a.  1 ml.                       c.  3 ml.
    b.  2 ml.                       d.  4 ml.

# CHAPTER 3

# Nursing Process in Drug Therapy

## True or false

_____ 1. When effective, it is generally better to use as few drugs in as low doses as possible.

_____ 2. Fixed-dose combinations of two or three drugs are preferred over two or three single drugs, when available.

_____ 3. Clients with severe renal disease often need smaller-than-average doses of drugs excreted by the kidney.

_____ 4. Many drugs can be given safely during pregnancy.

_____ 5. The preferred site for IM injection in infants is the thigh.

_____ 6. The most accurate method of calculating drug dosages for children is a method based on age.

_____ 7. Drug therapy in newborn infants must be very cautious because of immature liver and kidney functions.

_____ 8. Adverse drug effects are more likely to occur in elderly clients than in young or middle-aged adults.

_____ 9. Newer drugs are more effective than older ones.

_____ 10. The nurse should assess the client's condition before giving p.r.n. medications.

_____ 11. Drugs with long half-lives may not reach maximum therapeutic effect for several days or weeks.

_____ 12. Older adults have decreased amounts of body fat so fat-soluble drugs have a shorter duration of action.

_____ 13. Decreased serum protein levels can result in increased serum drug concentrations and increased risk of adverse effects.

_____ 14. When doing a medication history the nurse should also ask about non-prescription drug use including alcohol, caffeine, and nicotine.

_____ 15. A client's renal function should be considered before drug therapy is started.

## Review questions

1. M. is a 9-month-old placed on digoxin (Lanoxin) for symptoms of congestive heart failure. The dosage of this medication needs to be lower than that of a 2-year-old child because of M.'s
   a. immature blood-brain barrier.
   b. reduced liver enzymes.
   c. decreased glomerular filtration rate.
   d. lack of ability to metabolize drugs.

2. You are administering tetracycline to 3-year-old J. Before administering medication to J., you should
   a. ask him to identify himself.
   b. dilute the medication and put it in a syringe.
   c. place him on your lap.
   d. determine if the dosage is appropriate.

3. P. is a 5-year-old admitted with pneumonia and is to be started on IM injections of penicillin. Which of the following factors would be the most important when deciding where to administer the injection?

    a. P.'s height.
    b. P.'s body weight.

    c. P.'s age.
    d. P.'s mobility.

4. S., age 6, refuses to take her antibiotic. Identify your best response.

    a. "If you do not take the medication, your mother may not visit."
    b. "You may choose what you want to take with the medicine."

    c. "I will wait until your mother comes in."
    d. "I will come back in a little while."

5. The doctor orders a medication to be administered intramuscularly. The best location to administer the medication in a 4-month-old child is

    a. deltoid.
    b. vastus lateralis.

    c. gluteus maximus.
    d. dorsogluteal.

6. Which of the following statements is true about topical medications administered to pediatric clients?

    a. Infants absorb greater amounts of topical medications, which places them at greater risk for developing toxicity.
    b. Infants require greater amounts of topical medication because they have an elevated pH.

    c. Children should not receive topical medication in any form until after the age of 12.
    d. Children absorb less medication because of their decreased peripheral circulation.

7. Which of the following statements is true regarding the administration of fat-soluble medications in infants?

    a. A smaller portion of an infant's body is fat; therefore, the infant requires a smaller dose.
    b. A larger portion of an infant's body is fat; therefore, the infant requires a smaller dose.

    c. A smaller portion of an infant's body is fat; therefore, the infant requires a larger dose.
    d. A larger portion of an infant's body is fat; therefore, the infant requires a larger dose.

8. Mr. J., a 75-year-old client, has just received an initial dose of chlorpromazine (Thorazine). Because of his fat composition, you would expect that

    a. the onset of action of Thorazine will be rapid and the duration of effect will be prolonged.
    b. the onset of action of Thorazine will be prolonged and the duration of effect will be prolonged.

    c. the onset of action of Thorazine will be rapid and the duration of effect will be decreased.
    d. the onset of action of Thorazine will be prolonged and the duration of effect will be decreased.

9. Mr. B., an 89-year-old, has reduced hepatic functioning. Prior to administering medication, the nurse should be aware that this will

    a. reduce blood levels of certain drugs.
    b. increase the risk of drug toxicity.

    c. significantly limit the types of medications that can be administered.
    d. decrease the possibility of drug toxicity.

10. Which of the following statements by 93-year-old Mrs. S. leads you to believe that she has a potential problem with over-the-counter medications?

    a. "I take milk of magnesia every night before I go to sleep."
    b. "I take a vitamin pill every morning with my breakfast."

    c. "I use aspirin when I have arthritis pain."
    d. "I take Maalox when I eat Mexican food for the heartburn it causes me."

## Critical thinking case study

M., a 5-year-old, is admitted to your unit with a seizure disorder. M. weighs 44 lbs. Recommended dosage range of phenobarbital is 4–6 mg/kg/day for anticonvulsant effects.

1. Identify the maximum daily dosage.

2. If the above amount is to be given in three equal doses, what is the amount (mg) per dose?

3. The pharmacy sends you a phenobarbital solution containing 15 mg/ml. How many milliliters are needed for each dose calculated above?

M. is to be started on phenytoin (Dilantin). The recommended dosage range is 4–7 mg/kg/day. The pharmacy sends a solution of 100 mg/2 ml.

4. Identify the minimum daily dose (mg).

5. Identify the maximum daily dose (mg).

6. You are to administer two doses to M. daily. Identify the amount needed (ml) for each dose from a drug suspension with 30 mg/ml.

M. is complaining of pain. The physician orders 6 mg of morphine IM q6h. The recommended dosage range of morphine for a child is 0.1–0.2 mg/kg.

7. Identify where you would administer the medication.

8. Determine whether the dose ordered for M. is acceptable and discuss what you would do.

## Obtaining a medication history

Using the following form, select a patient, friend, or family member and obtain his or her medication history.

Name _____ Age _____
Occupation _____ Educational level _____

Health problems, acute and chronic

Do you have any allergies?

If yes, describe specific effects or symptoms.

## PART I. PRESCRIPTION MEDICATIONS

Do you take any prescription medications on a regular basis?

If yes, ask the following about each medication:

| | |
|---|---|
| Name | Dose |
| Frequency | Specific times |
| How long taken | Reason for use |

Are you able to take this medicine pretty much as prescribed?

What do you do when you miss a dose of medication?

Does anyone else help you take your medication?

What information or instructions were you given when the medication was first prescribed?

Do you think the medication is doing what it was prescribed to do?

Have you had any problems that you attribute to the medication?

Do you take any prescription medications on an irregular basis?

If yes, ask the following about each medication:

| | |
|---|---|
| Name | Reason |
| Dose | How long taken |
| Frequency | |

## PART II. NONPRESCRIPTION MEDICATIONS

Do you take any OTC medications for the following problems?

| PROBLEM | MEDICATION | | | |
|---|---|---|---|---|
| | Yes/No | Name | Amount | Frequency |
| Pain | | | | |
| Headache | | | | |
| Sleep | | | | |
| Cold | | | | |
| Indigestion | | | | |
| Heartburn | | | | |
| Diarrhea | | | | |
| Constipation | | | | |
| Other | | | | |

## PART III. SOCIAL HABITS

|  | Yes/No | Amount |
| --- | --- | --- |

Coffee (decaffeinated, regular)

Tea (decaffeinated, regular)

Soda (decaffeinated, regular, sugar-free)

Alcohol

Tobacco

Candy (chocolates, licorice, diet candy)

## PART IV PHYSICIANS

| Name | What you see them for | Phone # |
| --- | --- | --- |
| _____ | _____ | _____ |
| _____ | _____ | _____ |
| _____ | _____ | _____ |
| _____ | _____ | _____ |

# SECTION II

# Drugs Affecting the Central Nervous System

---

## CHAPTER 4

## Physiology of the Central Nervous System

---

## Complete the following sentences

1. The central nervous system is composed of a _____ and _____.

2. A _____ is a microscopic gap that separates _____.

3. Neurotransmitter substances include _____, _____(dopamine) (_____), _____, _____, _____, and _____.

4. The cerebral cortex is involved in all _____.

5. The thalamus receives impulses carrying sensations such as _____, _____, _____, and _____.

6. The hypothalamus regulates _____, _____, _____, and _____.

7. The medulla oblongata contains neurons that form the vital _____, _____, and _____ centers.

8. The reticular formation, when stimulated, produces _____.

9. The limbic system regulates _____ and _____.

10. The cerebellum coordinates _____. It also helps to _____ and _____.

11. Pyramidal tracts carry impulses from the brain to the spinal cord to the _____.

12. Extrapyramidal tracts do not enter the _____.

13. A lack of oxygen is called _____.

14. Hypoglycemia causes _____, _____, _____, _____, and _____.

15. _____ is required for the production and utilization of glucose.

16. A thiamine deficiency can cause degeneration of the _____ and can lead

    to _____ syndrome.

17. Moderate CNS depression produces _____, _____,

    _____, and _____.

18. Severe CNS depression produces _____, loss of reflexes,

    _____, and death.

19. Mild CNS stimulation produces _____, _____, and

    _____.

20. Moderate CNS stimulation produces _____,

    _____, and _____.

21. Excessive stimulation can cause _____, _____, and _____.

## Neurotransmission in the central nervous system

Neurotransmitter molecules, released by the presynaptic nerve, cross the synapse and bind with receptor proteins in the cell membrane of the postsynaptic nerve.

**Part A.** Identify the parts of Figure 4-1 by filling in the blanks with the correct terms below:

Receptor sites                    Postsynaptic nerve terminal
Neurotransmitters                 Synapse
Presynaptic nerve terminal        Release sites
Presynaptic nerve cell membrane   Postsynaptic nerve cell membrane

**Part B.** Complete the following statements by supplying the correct word or phrase.

1. _Norepinephrine_ is an excitatory neurotransmitter that affects mood and motor activity after crossing

   the _____ from the postganglionic sympathetic nervous system neurons and binding

   to _____ in the postsynaptic nerve cell membrane of the nerves

   that supply blood vessels to the adrenal medulla.

2. _Acetylcholine_ is an inhibitory neurotransmitter that exerts inhibitory effects on organs supplied by

   the vagus nerves by binding at _____.

## Review questions

1. Mr. J. has had a cerebral vascular accident (CVA) and he cries and laughs inappropriately. Which
   part of his brain was affected by the CVA?
   a. Limbic system.                    c. Cerebral cortex.
   b. Reticular formation network.      d. Cerebellum.

2. Thiamine is required for
   a. adequate cerebral blood flow.     c. production and utilization of glucose.
   b. cell metabolism.                  d. transference of nerve impulses.

3. Lack of this neurotransmitter substance causes Parkinson's disease.
   a. Acetylcholine.                    c. Serotonin.
   b. Dopamine.                         d. Endorphins.

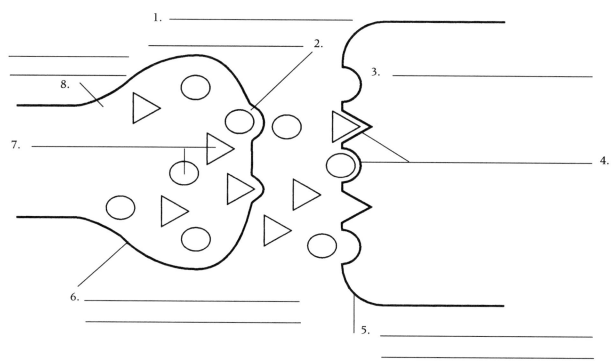

**Figure 4-1**

4. After neurosurgery, Mr. C. has an elevated temperature that is difficult to control with antipyretics. Swelling around which part of his brain is causing this problem?

   a. Thalamus.
   b. Cerebellum.

   c. Medulla oblongata.
   d. Hypothalamus.

5. Mrs. J., an insulin-dependent diabetic, is admitted with confusion. She has a blood sugar of 20 mg/dl, a potassium of 3.5 mEq/liter, and a $pO_2$ of 90 on admission. Her confusion is probably due to

   a. hypoxia.
   b. hypoglycemia.

   c. hypokalemia.
   d. thiamine deficiency.

6. Mild CNS stimulation can produce

   a. alertness.
   b. decreased perception of pain.

   c. insomnia.
   d. seizures.

7. When administering CNS depressants, one of the things the nurse must assess is

   a. hypoxia.
   b. bradycardia.

   c. adventitious lung sounds.
   d. respiratory depression.

8. The respiratory center is located in the

   a. limbic system.
   b. cerebellum.

   c. medulla oblongata.
   d. hypothalamus.

9. CNS stimulants are contraindicated in persons with a history of

   a. heart disease.
   b. Parkinsonism.

   c. diabetes mellitus.
   d. peptic ulcer disease.

10. After surgery, Mr. S.'s blood pressure drops. Which portion of the brain helps to regulate blood pressure?

   a. Medulla oblongata.
   b. Limbic system.

   c. Hypothalamus.
   d. Cerebrum.

# CHAPTER 5

# Narcotic Analgesics and Narcotic Antagonists

## Complete the following sentences

1. Depression of the CNS results in:
    a. _____.
    b. _____.
    c. _____.
    d. _____.
    e. _____.

2. Narcotics affect the GI system by _____ and causing _____.

3. Morphine sulfate can be administered _____, _____, and _____.

4. Roxanol _____/ml and MS Contin _____ tab/sustained release have been developed for cancer patients and can be given around the clock.

5. Codeine is often given with _____.

6. Meperidine hydrochloride (Demerol) differs from morphine in that it is _____ and produces _____. Usual doses of meperidine are _____ every _____ hrs.

7. Three examples of non-narcotic drugs used for moderate to severe pain are _____, _____, and _____.

8. A narcotic antagonist used to treat narcotic overdoses is _____.

9. Prior to administering pain medication a nurse should _____.

10. Besides the administration of pain medications, other nursing measures that can be employed include
    a. _____, b. apply _____, c. _____ techniques.

11. Three responses that a nurse must understand before administering pain medications are _____, _____, and _____.

12. The _____ route of administration is preferred when administering narcotics for acute pain because _____.

13. A _____ allows clients to self-administer pain medication.

14. Narcotics should not be used longer than _____ hrs. up to 72 hrs. except for malignant disease.

15. _____ is used with narcotic analgesics because of its spasm-preventing effects.

16. Infants may respond to pain by _____, _____, or with

 _____.

17. Before administering narcotics the nurse should check the client's _____ rate.

18. After pain medication has been administered, the client should be instructed not to _____

 or _____ without help.

19. Adverse reactions from pain medication include _____, _____,

 _____, _____, and constipation.

20. Persons taking pain medications should not drink _____.

## Word scramble

Unscramble the words, then circle them in the word find.

1. yatnfeln _____

2. cdeioen _____

3. ormdeel _____

4. dladdiiu _____

5. pimorhen _____

6. adtosl _____

7. ovardn _____

8. nbinua _____

9. craann _____

10. inwtal _____

**Word Find**

```
N O T H S B H Y P O F T I L C L C E F G H H J N K
K A D R E N E R G I C E N B E T A Z O L O L A N E
C M R I A S S A N L L X Q K E Z S V C D N C A T V
X Y Z T I P L D N E D R O N O N I R L A R N V R R
H L P O D I L A U D I D I C A Y Y O D A V V P P J
F N V A N L I C B R E E K X F H T G N A E S O S B
R I L U A A C A I D D U K L O E E U U E T O R R P
X T O S H R F R N O H A Z Y P X D K B B L K A O T
L R N A Y J R E C L N O S T Y H P E A N B E R E C
V A S G O N I Q P F E N T A N Y L K I S N L O K C
X T K X T G A A N G N P A P E C O R N I U O U S A
K J K X C Z A B T N T A D P V C D T E G F G X H O
V A S D I P I O C P R A O Z O I N J K A J K L D N
O N A E S O R P T I O N L W N C I N U C N C I V O
P T O M I I A N G I N Y B W I X K U N L S I N E T
A Z A E Y B I D L E S X F N I N S V D F H I A N I
R S C R F X Z Y N G R H V T G N J N A A E Z H T L
G E M O R P H I N E V K O N M H C H L O R Z I D E
Y N O L G D B P Q E R R O T V S P Q Y L O V B P C
L W I E F I C D L S N E V H O W G Y O Z A J O W D
F D O M R G G L I I S T P R O T E R E N E R Z N X
N C O E U M A D I N S F T P T M I G J F U W T C Y
E F D D Q C N Q N T A T D Y M N S J Z E B G O G C
```

## Review questions

1. Which of the following side effects from analgesics could potentially be life-threatening?

 a. Nausea and vomiting.

 b. Hypotension.

 c. Respiratory depression.

 d. Miosis.

2. You are caring for Mr. C. who is 2 days post-op and has been taking Demerol q4h. It is important to assess him for
   a. diarrhea.
   b. constipation.
   c. frequency.
   d. decreased urinary output.

3. Which of the following analgesics is commonly given with acetaminophen (Tylenol)?
   a. Codeine.
   b. Demerol.
   c. Morphine.
   d. Talwin.

4. An example of a non-narcotic analgesic used for moderate to severe pain is
   a. MS Contin.
   b. Tylenol.
   c. Roxanol.
   d. Nubain.

5. Prior to administering pain medication, you should always
   a. take the client to the bathroom.
   b. assess the level of pain.
   c. assess the client's blood pressure.
   d. assess the client's bowel sounds.

6. Mr. J. is admitted to the ER with an overdose of morphine. Which of the following drugs would be used to reverse the effects of the medication?
   a. Naloxone hydrochloride (Narcan).
   b. Butorphanol tartrate (Stadol).
   c. Buprenorphine (Buprenex).
   d. Nalbuphine hydrochloride (Nubain).

7. An expected side effect of opiates is
   a. pupillary constriction.
   b. pupillary dilation.
   c. dry mouth.
   d. difficulty in urinating.

8. Besides medications, other nursing actions that can be employed to reduce pain include all of the following *except*
   a. providing music.
   b. providing massage.
   c. ambulation.
   d. elevating lower extremities.

9. Which of the following statements by Mr. B. leads you to believe that he understands the teaching that you have done regarding pain medication?
   a. "I will only ask for medication if I am experiencing severe pain."
   b. "I cannot eat anything for 1 hour after I have had my pain medication."
   c. "If I want to smoke, I will call someone to stay with me."
   d. "No matter how bad the pain gets, I am not to ask for medication before 4 hours."

10. Which of the following symptoms would lead you to believe that an infant is experiencing pain?
    a. A pulse rate of 120.
    b. Muscle rigidity.
    c. A respiratory rate of 30.
    d. Cyanosis and apnea.

## Critical thinking case study

Your client, M.G., 29 years old, had a simple mastectomy 3 days ago. She has been receiving meperidine hydrochloride (Demerol) every 4 hours for pain since returning from surgery. At 11:30 this morning, when you helped her out of bed, she stated, "The medication makes me feel so much better."

1. Identify how you would respond to her statement.

2.  Describe the adverse effects you are assessing for.

While you are at lunch M.G. requests more pain medication and one of your colleagues administers it.

3.  Discuss what you would do when you return from lunch and find out M.G. has been medicated.

# CHAPTER 6

# Analgesic–Antipyretic–Anti-inflammatory and Related Drugs

## Matching exercise: terms and concepts

_____ 1. Toxic doses of this drug can cause liver necrosis.

_____ 2. This drug has antiplatelet properties.

_____ 3. The normal body response to tissue damage.

_____ 4. Substances found in body tissue that help regulate cell function.

_____ 5. A drug used in the treatment of gout.

_____ 6. A drug used only for the treatment of migraine headaches.

_____ 7. An ibuprofen drug available without a prescription.

_____ 8. A classic sign of an aspirin overdose.

_____ 9. A NSAID effective in the treatment of juvenile arthritis.

_____ 10. Bone marrow depression is an adverse effect of this drug.

A. Inflammation.

B. Ergotamine tartrate (Ergomar).

C. Ringing in the ears.

D. Acetaminophen (Tylenol).

E. Salicylic acid (ASA).

F. Naproxen (Naprosyn).

G. Advil.

H. Allopurinol (Zyloprim).

I. Prostaglandins.

J. Fever.

K. Headache.

L. Colchicine.

## True or false

_____ 1. Gangrene of the extremities has occurred after the administration of ergotamine tartrate (Ergomar).

_____ 2. Therapeutic effects from ergot preparations are usually evident within an hour after the drug is administered.

_____ 3. When diuretics are administered with allopurinol (Zyloprim), the effect of allopurinol (Zyloprim) is increased.

_____ 4. Persons taking indomethacin (Indocin) need to be assessed for confusion and drowsiness.

_____ 5. Clients receiving methysergide maleate (Sansert) should be examined frequently for pulmonary fibrosis and fibrotic thickening of cardiac valves and arteries.

## Review questions

1. Mr. T. is admitted with acute acetaminophen (Tylenol) poisoning. You should be assessing Mr. T. for
   a. neurotoxicity.
   b. renal failure.
   c. hepatoxicity.
   d. cardiac depression.

2. The physician asks you to get the antidote ready to administer to Mr. T. who has taken an overdose of acetaminophen (Tylenol). You will prepare
   a. acetylcysteine (Mucomyst).
   b. azathioprine (Imuran)
   c. hydroxychloroquine (Plaquenil).
   d. ascorbic acid.

3. Miss K., a 20-year-old college student with a history of asthma, is admitted to the college infirmary with dyspnea, bronchospasm, and a skin rash. Which of the following drugs could have precipitated her symptoms?
   a. Salicylic acid (aspirin).
   b. Acetaminophen (Tylenol).
   c. Ibuprofen (Motrin).
   d. Sulindac (Clinoril).

4. Miss B. calls the doctor's office because her daughter, age 3, has a high fever which she has not been able to bring down with acetaminophen (Tylenol). She wants to start her daughter on aspirin. Identify the best response to Mrs. B.
   a. Aspirin is not recommended because of its association with Reye's syndrome.
   b. You may give aspirin only if her temperature goes above 104°C.
   c. When aspirin and acetaminophen (Tylenol) are administered together, there is a greater risk of acetaminophen toxicity.
   d. Hypersensitivity to aspirin is common in children so we try to avoid using the drug whenever possible.

5. Which of the following statements by your client who is taking allopurinol (Zyloprim) leads you to believe that he has understood the teaching that you have done?
   a. "I will drink 2000–3000 ml per day."
   b. "I will drink cranberry juice to keep my urine acidic."
   c. "I will increase the protein in my diet."
   d. "I will limit my fluid intake to 1500 ml per day."

6. Mrs. B. takes aspirin four times per day for her arthritis. Which of the following statements by Mrs. B. leads you to believe that she is experiencing toxic side effects from the drug?
   a. "My heart seems to be beating fast."
   b. "I am very thirsty."
   c. "I have numbness and tingling in my legs."
   d. "I hear a roaring sound in my ears."

7. Mrs. G. is taking methysergide maleate (Sansert) for migraine headaches. Which of the following assessments should be done on a regular basis?
   a. Weight.
   b. WBC.
   c. Breath sounds.
   d. Blood sugar.

8. Drugs used in the treatment of gout should lower serum
   a. potassium levels.
   b. partial thromboplastin time.
   c. uric acid levels.
   d. urea nitrogen levels.

9. Mr. J. is started on colchicine for gouty arthritis. Mr. J. should be instructed to report which of the following side effects?
   a. Headache.
   b. Diarrhea.
   c. Fever.
   d. Itching.

10. Mr. J. is taking colchicine for acute gouty arthritis. He can expect to experience a therapeutic response after oral administration of the drug in
   a. 1–2 days.
   b. 3–4 days.
   c. 1 week.
   d. 2 weeks.

## Critical thinking case study

Mr. J. is a 55-year-old construction worker who has been prescribed indomethacin (Indocin) for rheumatoid arthritis which has been unresponsive to other drugs. In reviewing Mr. J.'s record, you find that he has a history of psychosis, diabetes, and hypertension.

1. Identify what in the client's history should be discussed with the physician before indomethacin (Indocin) is started and why.

2. Identify the periodic assessments that will be planned for this client.

3. Discuss the teaching you will do with this client.

The physician changes the prescribed medication to tolmetin (Tolectin).

4. Explain to the client the rationale for the change in medication.

# CHAPTER 7

# Sedative-Hypnotics

## Complete the following sentences

1. REM (_____) sleep is thought to be _____.

2. Insomnia is caused by _____, _____, _____, _____, and _____.

3. If barbiturates are used long term, they can produce a severe _____ when withdrawn.

4. Barbiturates stimulate liver cells to produce more _____ _____.

5. Barbiturates produce tolerance and lose their effectiveness in _____.

6. Barbiturates are contraindicated in _____, _____, _____, liver _____, _____, and acute intermittent porphyria.

7. Benzodiazepines should not be stopped abruptly after long-term use. They should be _____.

8. Chloral hydrate does not suppress _____. Tolerance to chloral hydrate develops in about _____.

9. Adverse effects of sedative-hypnotics include _____, _____, _____, _____, _____.

## True or false

_____ 1. Diphenhydramine (Benadryl), an antihistamine, can be used as a hypnotic.

_____ 2. Barbiturates can produce residual sedation or "morning hangover" which may last for several days after the drug is discontinued.

_____ 3. Long-acting benzodiazepines are more effective with the elderly.

_____ 4. A person experiencing withdrawal syndrome will experience confusion, depression, and weight loss.

_____ 5. Sedative-hypnotics increase REM sleep.

_____ 6. When barbiturates are administered with phenytoin (Dilantin) the dosage of Dilantin needs to be decreased.

_____ 7. Sedative-hypnotics lose their effectiveness in 2–4 weeks if taken nightly and can cause sleep disturbances when withdrawn.

## Review questions

1. Ms. H. is started on pentobarbital (Nembutal) because of insomnia. Which of the following statements by Ms. H. would lead you to believe that she understands the teaching that you have done?
   a. "I must never take the medication before 11 p.m."
   b. "The medication will be effective for about 2 weeks."
   c. "In low doses, you can use this medication for up to 1 year."
   d. "I will take the medication an hour before I plan on going to bed."

2. Mr. H., who is taking amobarbital sodium (Amytal), complains of feeling tired in the morning. What should you tell him?
   a. "You should stop the medication and not take it anymore."
   b. "This is a common side effect with this medication and may last several days after the drug is discontinued."
   c. "This is a common side effect and it will subside in a few days."
   d. "If you begin to experience anxiety, restlessness, or tremors, then contact your physician."

3. An antihistamine that can also be used as a hypnotic is
   a. diphenhydramine (Benadryl).
   b. flurazepam (Dalmane).
   c. chloral hydrate.
   d. temazepam (Restoril).

4. Which of the following would promote sleep?
   a. Increase calcium in diet.
   b. Decrease exercise.
   c. Increase caffeine-containing beverages during the day.
   d. Decrease fluid intake at night.

5. When barbiturates are abruptly discontinued, this could pose a risk of
   a. confusion.
   b. depression.
   c. hypertension.
   d. seizures.

6. The use of barbiturates is contraindicated in persons with a history of
   a. diabetes.
   b. epilepsy.
   c. alcohol abuse.
   d. mental illness.

7. Which of the following is an intermediate-acting barbiturate?
   a. Pentobarbital (Nembutal).
   b. Secobarbital (Seconal).
   c. Amobarbital (Amytal).
   d. Phenobarbital (Luminal).

8. In comparing sedative-hypnotics the following is true:
   a. Chloral hydrate does not produce drowsiness and will not cause physical dependence, but barbiturates will.
   b. Barbiturates and benzodiazepines are equal in suppressing REM sleep.
   c. Barbiturates are less likely to produce drowsiness than benzodiazepines.
   d. Benzodiazepines are less likely to cause dependence and abuse than barbiturates.

9. Mr. J. receives flurazepam (Dalmane) at bedtime. The desired effect will be seen within
   a. 10 minutes.
   b. 30 minutes.
   c. 60 minutes.
   d. 70 minutes.

10. When barbiturates are ordered to be administered with phenytoin (Dilantin),
    a. a larger dose may be required because of increased metabolism.
    b. a smaller dose may be required because of decreased metabolism.
    c. there needs to be no change in the dose.
    d. there is a problem because these two drugs cannot be administered together.

## Critical thinking case study

You are admitting Mr. Z. for removal of a bladder tumor in the morning. When you are filling out the admission questionnaire, you discover that Mr. Z. has been taking over-the-counter sleeping aids for several months and a week ago he began doubling the dose. Mr. Z. expresses concern that he will not be able to sleep in the hospital.

1. Identify how you will respond to Mr. Z.'s concern.

2. Discuss alternatives to medication that can help him sleep.

The physician orders flurazepam (Dalmane) the evening before surgery. Mr. Z. awakes feeling lethargic.

3. Suggest an alternative to the physician that may be appropriate for Mr. Z.

4. Identify two possible nursing diagnoses for Mr. Z.

# CHAPTER 8

# Antianxiety Drugs

## Complete the following sentences

1. When anxiety is _____, it impairs the ability to function.

2. The classification of anxiety disorder includes _____ and _____, _____, _____, _____, and _____.

3. Symptoms of anxiety are related to _____, _____, and _____.

4. The _____ are the most commonly used drugs for situational anxiety.

5. Benzodiazepines cause _____ and _____ dependence.

6. Benzodiazepines are _____ soluble and bound to _____.

7. Chlordiazepoxide (_____), diazepam (_____), and clorazepate (_____) have _____ half-lives and require _____ days to reach a steady state.

8. Benzodiazepines are used as _____, _____, and _____ agents. They are also used for _____ and to prevent _____ and _____ in acute alcohol withdrawal and as muscle relaxants.

9. Benzodiazepines are contraindicated in _____, _____, _____, and _____.

10. Buspirone (_____) causes less _____ and does not cause _____ or _____ dependence but lacks the _____ and _____ effects of benzodiazepines.

11. When hydroxyzine (_____) is combined with narcotic analgesics, it _____ their sedative effects.

12. Hydroxyzine has _____ and _____ effects.

13. Meprobamate (Equanil, Miltown) can cause _____, _____, _____, and _____ with long-term use.

14. Short-acting benzodiazepines are usually given in _____ daily doses.

15. Clinical manifestations of withdrawal syndrome include _____, _____, _____, _____, _____, and _____. More serious manifestations include _____, _____, _____, and _____.

16. In the presence of liver disease, the benzodiazepines of choice are _____ (_____)
    and _____ (_____).

17. When giving diazepam (Valium) IV, you should inject at the rate of _____ and use a
    _____ vein and have _____ available.

18. Drugs that increase effects of antianxiety agents include _____, antidepressants, _____,
    _____, _____, _____, _____, and _____.

19. Drugs that decrease effects of antianxiety agents include _____, _____,
    _____, _____, and caffeine.

## Nursing diagnosis

Identify three possible nursing diagnoses, pertinent assessment data, and nursing interventions for persons requiring antianxiety medications.

| Nursing Diagnoses | Assessment | Nursing Interventions |
| --- | --- | --- |
| 1. | | |
| 2. | | |
| 3. | | |

**DEFINE:**

ANXIETY

## Review questions

1. Mr. H., a 76-year-old man in a long-term care facility, is to be started on meprobamate (Equanil). The nursing goal that would be a priority for Mr. H. is that the
   a. client will feel more calm and relaxed.
   b. client will verbalize a reduction in anxiety.
   c. client will have an adequate fluid intake.
   d. client will be free of falls or injury.

2. Which of the following statements by Mrs. G., who is to be started on diazepam (Valium), would lead you to believe that she needs additional instruction?

   a. "I will not drink alcohol or caffeine."
   b. "I will not drive once I have started the medicine."
   c. "I know that this medication should only be taken for a short time."
   d. "If I become drowsy, I will stop the medication."

3. Which one of the following clients exhibits a therapeutic response to alprazolam (Xanax)?

   a. Mr. J. works in his yard.
   b. Mrs. A. naps during the day and sleeps at night.
   c. Mrs. J. talks to her children on the phone.
   d. Mrs. H. eats three meals a day.

4. Miss P., a 29-year-old female, is admitted with withdrawal syndrome secondary to abruptly discontinuing clorazepate (Tranxene) 30 mg t.i.d. She is anxious and complains of a headache and palpitations. The measures that should be instituted when Miss P. arrives on your unit include

   a. monitoring vital signs q2h.
   b. providing one-on-one continuous supervision.
   c. keeping client NPO.
   d. providing a private room with minimal stimulation.

5. If Mrs. H. appears sedated when a dose of lorazepam (Ativan) is due, you should

   a. omit the dose and record the reason.
   b. delay the dose and try to stimulate the client.
   c. call the physician immediately.
   d. give the dose because the sedation is only temporary.

6. You are to administer diazepam (Valium) 10 mg IV push for a 16-year-old with epilepsy who is actively seizing. What should you be observing for?

   a. Bradycardia.
   b. Apnea.
   c. Hypertension.
   d. Increased seizure activity.

7. The order reads: administer meperidine (Demerol) 50 mg IM, hydroxyzine (Vistaril) 25 mg IM, and atropine 0.25 mg. Can these medications be administered together?

   a. They must all be administered separately.
   b. Demerol and Vistaril can be given together.
   c. Demerol and atropine can be given together.
   d. All the medications can be administered in the same syringe.

8. The physician's order reads: meperidine (Demerol) 25 mg and hydroxyzine (Vistaril) 25 mg IM. Demerol comes in 50 mg/1 cc and Vistaril comes in 100 mg/2 cc. What is the total amount of solution that you will be administering?

   a. 0.5 ml.
   b. 0.75 ml.
   c. 1 ml.
   d. 1.5 ml.

9. When administering diazepam (Valium) IM, the best location to administer it in is

   a. arm (deltoid).
   b. leg (vastus lateralis)
   c. hip (gluteus maximus).
   d. all of the above.

10. Mrs. J. is to be started on buspirone (BuSpar). Which of the following instructions would it be important to give to Mrs. J.?

    a. "It may take a few weeks before you experience the full effect of this medication."
    b. "You will begin to experience a decrease in your anxiety in one week."
    c. "If you notice a sore throat or experience alopecia, contact your physician."
    d. "Vomiting and diarrhea are common side effects of the drug; stop the medication if you experience these side effects."

## Critical thinking case study

Mr. J. is admitted to your unit with a diagnosis of gastritis. He is currently taking Prolixin 1 mg t.i.d. lanoxin (Digoxin) 0.25 mg q.d. and furosemide (Lasix) 40 mg b.i.d. Mr. J.'s physician orders cimetadine (Tagamet) 300 mg q.i.d. Forty-eight hours after admission, Mr. J. becomes agitated. Before you are able to contact the physician, Mr. J. has a seizure.

  1.  Identify and prioritize your nursing actions.

The physician orders Valium, 10 mg IV push.

  2.  Identify why Valium was ordered and whether the dose falls within the therapeutic range.

Valium comes in a vial that states: add 1.8 ml of solution. The total amount of solution in the vial after dilution is 2 ml which contains 10 mg of Valium.

  3.  Identify how many milliliters you will administer per minute.

  4.  Describe what you will be assessing for.

Once Mr. J.'s seizures have subsided, the physician orders chlordiazepoxide (Librium) 100 mg q8h PO.

  5.  Identify the potential adverse reactions and appropriate nursing measures.

# CHAPTER 9

# Antipsychotic Drugs

## Complete the following sentences

1. _____ is the most common functional psychosis.

2. The most frequently used group of antipsychotic drugs is the _____.

3. Phenothiazines exert many pharmacologic effects including _____,

   _____, _____,

   _____, and _____.

4. Antipsychotic drugs decrease the effects of _____.

5. Antipsychotic drugs decrease hyperarousal symptoms which include _____,

   _____, _____, _____, _____,

   _____, and delusions.

6. Clinical indications for the use of antipsychotics not associated with psychiatric illness include

   treatment of _____ and _____ and intractable hiccups.

7. Place a *ca* next to the conditions in which antipsychotic medications should be used with caution
   and a *ci* next to the conditions in which the use of antipsychotics is contraindicated.

   a. Liver damage _____.

   b. Coronary artery disease _____.

   c. CVA _____.

   d. Seizure disorders _____.

   e. Diabetes mellitus _____.

   f. Parkinson's disease _____.

   g. Glaucoma _____.

   h. Peptic ulcer disease _____.

   i. Bone marrow depression _____.

   j. Hypertension _____.

   k. Chronic respiratory disorders _____.

   l. Severely depressive states _____.

   m. Coma _____.

8. Chlorprothixene (_____) and thiothixene (_____) are used for their _____ effects.

9. Haloperidol (_____) produces a _____ incidence of _____ and _____ and a _____ incidence of _____.

10. Haldol is also used in _____, _____, and _____.

11. Loxapine (_____) and clozapine (_____) are used for the treatment of schizophrenia. Clozapine has a high risk of _____ and other adverse effects including _____, _____, and ECG changes.

12. Pimozide (Orap) is used for the treatment of _____. Serious adverse effects include _____, _____, and _____.

13. Goals of treatment with antipsychotic drugs are to _____, _____, and _____.

14. Some clients who do not respond well to one type of antipsychotic drug may _____. If a substitution of a new drug is necessary, the old drug should be decreased while substituting _____ doses of the new drug.

15. Clients who are unable or unwilling to take daily doses of antipsychotic drugs may be given _____ of _____ (_____).

16. The best time to administer antipsychotic drugs is _____ daily within _____ bedtime.

17. Liquid concentrates should be mixed with _____ of _____.

18. Antiadrenergic effects include _____, _____, _____, _____, and _____.

19. Anticholinergic effects include _____, dental _____, _____, _____, _____, and _____.

20. Endocrine effects include _____, _____, and _____; and in males, _____.

## Word scramble

Fill in the trade name next to the generic name, then circle the trade name in the word find.

1. acetophenazine _____

2. thioridazine _____

3. prochlorperazine _____

4. fluphenazine hydrochloride

   _____

5. chlorpromazine _____

6. perphenazine _____

7. promazine _____

8. trifluoperazine _____

9. molindone _____

10. pimozide _____

11. clozapine _____

12. haloperidol _____

13. chlorprothixene _____

14. thiothixene _____

15. loxapine _____

**Word Find**

```
T A L E F D F D Q C N Q N S P A R I N E T X A T W
A N C O E K N U M O A R D I Q N B P N T P T M I H
R G P T M T M I G J F U W T C Y I I D E O M R G K
A G G L I I S T M N P K R O T E Z R E N R E Z N X
C L L W I N E F I C D E L S N A X U O W Y O Z A R
T Y O N R D G S D B P W B R P R O T V S P Q V Y L
A V G E M A A O R H P H I M E V K O F N M H T M I
N Z R B T L C L O I X M O B A N I X E U Z Y R N G
R H V T G H F J J N A C L O Z A R I L E A Z I H O
A T L Y A Z O Y B I D L E S P X T F N D N S L S V
D F H I M D F R U T P T O R T I D S H L B Z A T E
X O N A B Q S O A R P P T I U O N D C O W N F C I
R U C N K I V O V Z A S H Q O I P C P X R A O L Z
F K J K Z X C Z A M I B T A N D A O A I P V N C D
G C D T X E C F J G E N F G L X H O L T E B T M O
C D T I P B Q T U D H L E R A D P D A A P X D A T
P L A A W S M A X V T G L A A G O N P N A P E C N
O R R N I U O Q U S P U S A V A S L G E O N E I Q
P O F E J N T N A N Y L K I R S B N C L K I S N L
O K C P L V R N A I A Y J R E I C L N O S W T Y H
P E A R B S E R E V C X T S T E L A Z I N E T O S
P R O L I X I N X A A S O N I Q U G P E N T A N Y
L K I S N G L O O K L N R N A Y J R E C L I N O S
T Y H P E A M B E R E C E P X T O S H R F R N O H
H M A Z Y P X D R M B B L K A O T R I L U A A C B
```

## Review questions

1. Which of the following behaviors would indicate a positive response to the antipsychotic medication?
   a. Feeding self.
   b. Sleeping at night.
   c. Participating in self-care activities.
   d. Pacing back and forth.

2. Mr. H. has been started on fluphenazine hydrochloride (Prolixin). Which of these statements by the client indicates that he understands the instructions?
   a. "My symptoms can reoccur if I do not take my medication regularly."
   b. "If I feel extremely tired, I should stop the medication."
   c. "If I begin to feel better, I will still need to take the medication, but I will no longer need counseling."
   d. "I will limit my physical activity to one hour a day."

3. Six weeks after starting chlorpromazine (Thorazine), Mrs. P. complains of difficulty chewing and swallowing. These symptoms may be the result of

   a. akathesia.
   b. epilepsy.
   c. dykinesias.
   d. dystonias.

4. Mr. H., a 79-year-old nursing home resident, is started on thioridazine (Mellaril) for psychosis. Which of the following would Mr. H. be at high risk for?

   a. Injury related to excessive sedation and movement disorders.
   b. Altered bowel elimination; diarrhea.
   c. Altered tissue perfusion related to hypertension.
   d. Nutritional deficit related to weight loss.

5. Antipsychotic drugs are contraindicated in persons with

   a. renal disease.
   b. Parkinson's disease.
   c. senile dementia.
   d. Alzheimer's disease.

6. Which of the following statements is true with regard to drug interactions with antipsychotics? Antipsychotics, when taken with

   a. thiazide diuretics, can produce hypertension.
   b. antihistamines, can produce increased agitation.
   c. antacids, can produce gastric irritation and diarrhea.
   d. CNS depressants, can produce seizures.

7. Mrs. C. has been started on perphenazine (Trilafon). Which of these statements by the client indicates she needs additional instructions?

   a. "I will see the dentist every 6 months and brush my teeth frequently."
   b. "I will only go outside at night."
   c. "If I get dizzy, I will not try to stand or walk."
   d. "I will not take antacids with my medication."

8. When doing discharge teaching with Mr. C., who is taking clozapine (Clozaril), all of the following instructions are appropriate. Which one is the most important?

   a. "You need to see the doctor weekly to have a white blood count done."
   b. "You should have your blood pressure checked monthly."
   c. "A diet high in fiber with a good fluid intake will help you maintain normal bowel habits."
   d. "Chewing sugarless gum will help your dry mouth."

9. Mr. H., who is taking antipsychotic medication, complains of muscular rigidity, shuffling gait, hypersalivation, and drooling. Based on these findings the nurse should suspect

   a. increased psychosis.
   b. dystonia.
   c. tardive dyskinesia.
   d. Parkinsonism.

10. After assessing Mrs. J., who has just been admitted to your unit, you obtain the following data: BP 86/50, pulse 58, respirations 16, weight loss of 5 lbs. Because Mrs. J. is taking promazine (Sparine), which one of these findings should be reported?

    a. Blood pressure.
    b. Pulse.
    c. Respirations.
    d. Weight loss.

## Critical thinking case study

Mr. P., an 89-year-old, is admitted from home with a diagnosis of psychosis. He is agitated and combative. The following laboratory tests are ordered: SGOT, WBC, Na+, K+, Cl−, glucose.

1. Identify medical conditions in which the use of antipsychotic medications would be contraindicated.

Mr. P. is started on fluphenazine hydrochloride (Prolixin) IM.

2. Determine what an appropriate dose for Mr. P. would be and discuss how you came to your conclusion.

Mr. P.'s daughter is very concerned about him and asks when she can expect to see improvement in his condition.

3. Discuss your response to Mr. P.'s daughter.

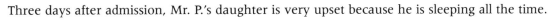

Three days after admission, Mr. P.'s daughter is very upset because he is sleeping all the time.

4. Explain to Mr. P.'s daughter what she can expect.

One month after admission, Mr. P. develops compulsive involuntary restless movements. Mr. P.'s daughter questions whether the psychosis has returned.

5. Describe your response to Mr. P.'s daughter.

Mr. P.'s daughter plans on taking him home to live with her.

6. Discuss what instructions she should be given.

# CHAPTER **10**

# **Antidepressants**

## Complete the following sentences

1. Symptoms of depression include:

   a. _____.

   b. _____.

   c. _____.

   d. _____.

   e. _____.

   f. _____.

   g. _____.

   h. _____.

   i. _____.

2. Secondary depression may be precipitated by _____, _____, or _____.

3. Tricyclic antidepressants produce _____ _____and cardiac dysrhythmias.

4. Fluoxetine (_____) produces common adverse effects including _____, _____, _____, and _____.

5. Monoamine oxidase inhibitors may interact with _____ and _____ to produce _____.

6. Foods that interact with monoamine oxidase inhibitors are those containing _____.

7. Identify eight commonly eaten foods that are high in tyramine.

   a. _____.          e. _____.

   b. _____.          f. _____.

   c. _____.          g. _____.

   d. _____.          h. _____.

8. Lithium carbonate (_____) is used for clients with _____.

9. _____ is a prerequisite for lithium therapy.

10. Deviations in serum _____ affect lithium levels.

11. Monoamine oxidase inhibitors are given for _____.

12. Lithium may be given for _____.

13. A therapeutic effect from TCAs is expected in _____ weeks.

14. For most clients the therapeutic serum level for lithium is _____ mEq/l.

15. The choice of an antidepressant depends upon the _____ of depression and its _____.

16. Common adverse effects from TCAs seen when treatment is initiated include: _____,

    _____, _____, _____, _____,

    _____, _____, and _____ sweating.

17. Adverse effects occurring at higher serum drug levels include: _____, _____,

    _____, _____, _____, _____,

    _____, _____, _____, and _____.

## Sentence correction

Circle the word(s) that make the sentence incorrect and place the correct word(s) in the space provided.

_____ 1. An adverse effect of antidepressants that is useful in treating enuresis is insomnia.

_____ 2. Furosemide (Lasix) should not be administered with MAO inhibitors because a hypertensive crisis could occur.

_____ 3. A deficiency of potassium increases the risk of lithium toxicity.

_____ 4. Fluoxetine (Prozac) needs to be administered b.i.d.

_____ 5. Blurred vision should be reported to the physician for persons taking MAO inhibitors.

_____ 6. Adequate hepatic function is a prerequisite for lithium therapy.

_____ 7. Depression results from a deficiency of dopamine and acetylcholine.

_____ 8. Tricyclic antidepressants produce a relatively high incidence of cardiac failure.

_____ 9. For severe lithium overdose, gastric lavage is the preferred treatment.

_____10. Caffeine decreases the effects of tricyclic antidepressants.

_____11. If therapeutic effects from TCAs are not seen in 8 weeks, the medication should be discontinued.

_____12. Lithium is used to control severe depression.

_____13. Diazepam (Valium) is used to reverse anticholinergic effects of TCAs.

_____14. Serum lithium levels should be drawn every 6 months.

_____15. TCAs are not recommended for persons under the age of 18 except for treatment of enuresis; then they may be used in children over age 12.

## Review questions

1. Mr. H. is started on amitriptyline (Elavil). Which of the following statements by Mr. H. leads you to believe that he understands the teaching you have done?
   a. "I will need to take the medication for 2–3 weeks."
   b. "I will need to take the medication until my symptoms subside."
   c. "I will take the medication for several months."
   d. "I will take the medication the rest of my life."

2. Which of the following electrolytes must be maintained at a steady state when a person is taking lithium?
   a. Sodium.
   b. Potassium.
   c. Chloride.
   d. Magnesium.

3. Foods that should be avoided when a person is taking MAO inhibitors include
   a. citrus fruits.
   b. dark green vegetables.
   c. caffeine and chocolate.
   d. red meat.

4. Mr. A. is admitted to your unit with a diagnosis of overdose of doxepin (Sinequan). Which of the following nursing diagnoses would be a priority?
   a. High risk for injury related to sedation.
   b. Knowledge deficit related to effects and usage of antidepressants.
   c. Sleep pattern disturbances related to depression.
   d. High risk for decreased cardiac output related to cardiac dysrhythmias and hypotension.

5. Mr. J. is admitted with bipolar affective disorder and is to be started on lithium. Mr. J. is taking prednisone, digoxin (Lanoxin), insulin, and theophylline. Which medication that the client is taking would you make the physician aware of before you start the lithium?
   a. Prednisone.
   b. Lanoxin.
   c. Insulin.
   d. Theophylline.

6. Which of the following statements by your client, who is being discharged on a TCA, would lead you to believe that he does not understand the discharge instructions?
   a. "I can drink small amounts of alcohol and it will not cause any problems."
   b. "I will stop smoking cigarettes."
   c. "I will check with the pharmacist before I buy any over-the-counter medications."
   d. "I will tell my dentist before he gives me any medications that I am taking an antidepressant."

7. Mr. P.'s family asks you when they can expect to see a therapeutic response to the antidepressant medication. Your best response would be
   a. 24–48 hours.
   b. 7–10 days.
   c. 2–3 weeks.
   d. 6–8 weeks.

8. Mrs. H., a 38-year-old accountant, is to be started on phenelzine (Nardil), an MAO inhibitor. Which of the following should be monitored frequently?
   a. Blood pressure.
   b. Blood sugar.
   c. Weight.
   d. Hemoglobin.

9. You are giving Mr. J. instructions prior to his being discharged on isocarboxazid (Marplan), an MAO inhibitor. You should tell him that if he ingests foods high in tyramine, the following can occur:
   a. Nausea, vomiting, and diarrhea.
   b. Orthostatic hypotension.
   c. Hypertensive crisis.
   d. Hallucinations.

10. R.S. was admitted with agitation and hyperactivity related to bipolar affective disorder. After 5 days of treatment with lithium, he complains of feeling slowed down and has increased thirst but remains hyperactive. Your analysis is that
    a. your client remains manic but has developed toxic side effects from lithium.
    b. your client remains manic without serious side effects of toxicity.
    c. the treatment has been ineffective; he should be calm at this time.
    d. a higher dose is required to achieve a therapeutic effect.

## Critical thinking case study

Mr. J. is a 76-year-old male admitted to your unit with a diagnosis of depression.

1.  Discuss how the diagnosis of depression is made.

Mr. J. has a history of diabetes, gout, chronic obstructive pulmonary disease, and allergies to pollen and animal dander.

2.  Identify which of Mr. J.'s illnesses need to be considered before prescribing antidepressants and discuss why.

The physician starts Mr. J. on doxepin (Sinequan).

3.  Identify appropriate goals for Mr. J.

4.  Specify what information Mr. J. should be given before going home.

Mr. J. returns to the clinic 3 weeks after starting antidepressant therapy, complaining of fatigue and lethargy. Mr. J. states that he is feeling worse and does not want to continue the medication.

5. Identify the assessments you will do.

6. Discuss how you will deal with Mr. J.'s refusal to continue the medication.

# CHAPTER 11

# Anticonvulsants

## Complete the following sentences

1. A seizure is a _____
   _____.

2. A convulsion is a _____
   _____.

3. Epilepsy is a _____.

4. Epilepsy is diagnosed with an _____.

5. When epilepsy begins in infancy, it is caused by _____, _____
   _____, or _____.

6. Phenobarbital may be used alone especially in _____. Often it is used in combination
   with _____ (Dilantin) when seizure activity is not adequately controlled.

7. A therapeutic Dilantin level is _____/ml.

8. Diazepam (_____) is used to terminate _____ _____.

9. _____ (Tegretol) is used for clients whose seizures
   _____. Carbamazepine is also
   used to treat facial pain associated with _____.

10. The six following things may produce seizures in people who have not had a previous history of
    seizures: _____, _____, hypoxia, hypoglycemia,
    _____, and withdrawal from CNS depressants.

11. For most clients anticonvulsant therapy is _____.

12. Discontinuing or changing antiseizure drugs must be done over
    _____.

13. If phenytoin (Dilantin) is given intravenously, the intravenous line must be flushed before and
    after with _____ because if phenytoin (Dilantin) mixes with a dextrose solution it
    will_____.

14. If phenytoin (Dilantin) is administered too rapidly, it may produce
    _____, _____, cardiac _____,
    and _____.

15. Many anticonvulsants decrease levels of _____, which can lead to megaloblastic anemia.

## True or false

_____ 1. An overdose of lidocaine can produce seizures.

_____ 2. During a seizure, a spoon should be inserted between the teeth to protect the tongue.

_____ 3. Tonic-clonic seizures can result in agnosia which lasts 3–4 hours after the seizure is over.

_____ 4. Most anticonvulsant drugs have the potential for causing blood, liver, and kidney disorders.

_____ 5. Oral anticonvulsants should be administered on an empty stomach.

_____ 6. Alcohol increases the effect of phenytoin (Dilantin).

_____ 7. Skin disorders are common with almost all anticonvulsant drugs.

## Crossword puzzle

### Across

2. Patients can build up a tolerance to this drug with long-term use.
4. A benzodiazepine used for acute alcohol withdrawal and to manage partial seizures.
5. The drug of choice for treating status epilepticus.
9. One of the safest, most effective, most widely used anticonvulsants.

### Down

1. A type of seizure characterized by spasmodic reactions.
3. May cause life-threatening blood dyscrasia.
6. The initial drug of choice in adults who are experiencing tonic-clonic seizures.
7. Used to treat absence and mixed seizures.
8. A brain disorder that causes seizures.
10. Used to terminate acute seizures.

## Review questions

1. Mrs. H., a 48-year-old diabetic, has just been admitted to the emergency room because of a seizure. Since Mrs. H. is not an epileptic, identify a possible cause for the seizure.
   a. Hypoglycemia.
   b. Hyperglycemia.
   c. Acidosis.
   d. Anaphylactic reaction.

2. The drug of choice for treating generalized seizures in adults is
   a. ethosuximide (Zarontin).
   b. clonazepam (Klonopin).
   c. phenytoin (Dilantin).
   d. diazepam (Valium).

3. A therapeutic phenytoin (Dilantin) serum level is
   a. 2–7 µg/ml.
   b. 10–20 µg/ml.
   c. 25–30 µg/ml.
   d. 40–50 µg/ml.

4. Mrs. J. is admitted with trigeminal neuralgia. Which of the following drugs would be most effective in treating her facial pain?

   a. Carbamazepine (Tegretol).

   b. Clonazepam (Klonopin).

   c. Phenobarbital.

   d. Ethosuximide (Zarontin).

5. Prior to administering phenytoin (Dilantin) intravenously you must

   a. check the client's blood pressure.

   b. flush the line with normal saline.

   c. administer phenobarbital.

   d. attach the client to a cardiac monitor.

6. Administration of anticonvulsants for long periods can produce megaloblastic anemia because of decreased levels of

   a. ascorbic acid.

   b. thiamine.

   c. vitamin $B_{12}$.

   d. folic acid.

7. The dosage of phenytoin (Dilantin) may need to be adjusted if your client is taking

   a. diuretics.

   b. antidepressants.

   c. oral antidiabetic agents.

   d. bronchodilators.

8. Which of the following statements by Mr. S. would lead you to believe that he understands his discharge instructions about anticonvulsant therapy?

   a. "I need to take good care of my teeth and gums."

   b. "I should take the medication on an empty stomach."

   c. "Once my seizures are under control, I will no longer need the medication."

   d. "I can drink alcohol and it will not affect my medication."

9. The drug of choice for status epilepticus is

   a. ethosuximide (Zarontin).

   b. clonazepam (Klonopin).

   c. phenytoin (Dilantin).

   d. diazepam (Valium).

10. Persons taking carbamazepine (Tegretol) must be observed for

   a. hypertension.

   b. weight gain.

   c. night blindness.

   d. blood dyscrasia.

## Critical thinking case study

C.M., a 12-year-old girl, has been admitted to your unit with a head injury. She has been having intermittent seizures since her hospitalization 24 hours ago. (Learners may need to use additional sources to answer these questions.)

1. Describe how you will respond if C.M. has another seizure.

The physician prescribes phenytoin (Dilantin) and phenobarbital for C.M.

2. Compare the adverse effects of phenytoin (Dilantin) and phenobarbital.

C.M.'s mom asks you if she will have to take the medication the rest of her life.

3. Describe your response.

C.M. is discharged on phenytoin (Dilantin) and phenobarbital.

4. Identify the teaching that you will do prior to discharge.

# CHAPTER 12

# Anti-Parkinson Drugs

## Complete the following sentences

1. Parkinson's disease is a _____, _____, _____, disorder of the CNS character-ized by _____ _____, _____.

2. People with Parkinson's disease have a decrease in _____ and an increase in _____.

3. Dopaminergic drugs that exert beneficial effects in Parkinson's disease are _____(Dopar), carbidopa (_____), amantadine (_____), and bromocriptine (_____).

4. Amantadine (_____) increases _____.

5. Bromocriptine (_____) stimulates _____ _____.

6. Anticholinergic drugs are contraindicated in clients with _____, _____, _____, urinary bladder _____, and _____.

7. Levodopa (Larodopa, Dopar) is the _____ drug available for the treatment of Parkinson's disease.

8. With long-term use of levodopa (Dopar), clients experience _____ of Parkinsonism symptoms.

9. A levodopa-carbidopa combination product is (_____) which allows more levodopa to reach the _____.

10. Amantadine (_____) relieves Parkinsonism symptoms in _____ days, but loses its effectiveness in 6–8 weeks of continuous administration.

11. Bromocriptine (_____) may _____of levodopa and reduce the _____.

12. Levodopa is the drug of choice when _____ are the prominent symptoms.

## True or false

_____ 1. Levodopa (Dopar) and bromocriptine (Parlodel) should be given on an empty stomach.

_____ 2. Anticholinergic drugs produce atropine-like effects.

_____ 3. Dyskinesia is a side effect of levodopa and results in involuntary movements of the tongue, mouth, face, or whole body.

_____ 4. Persons taking levodopa should be observed for bradycardia.

_____ 5. Bromocriptine (Parlodel) can produce a patchy blue discoloration on skin on the legs called livedo reticularis.

_____ 6. Persons taking levodopa need to increase their intake of protein and vitamin $B_6$.

## Review questions

1. Mr. J. is to go home on levodopa (Dopar). Which of the following statements by Mr. J. leads you to believe that he has understood the teaching that you have done?
   a. "I will avoid all beverages containing caffeine."
   b. "I will eat no citrus fruits."
   c. "I will eat no green leafy vegetables."
   d. "I will not eat foods high in vitamin B$_6$."

2. Livedo reticularis is an adverse sign associated with the use of
   a. levodopa (Dopar).
   b. bromocriptine (Parlodel).
   c. amantadine (Symmetrel).
   c. carbidopa (Lodosyn).

3. Levodopa is contraindicated in persons who have
   a. diabetes mellitus.
   b. peptic ulcer disease.
   c. arthritis.
   d. heart disease.

4. Which of the following is an adverse effect from levodopa?
   a. Dyskinesia.
   b. Constipation.
   c. Hypertension.
   d. Seizure.

5. Which of the following is an adverse effect from anticholinergic therapy?
   a. Bradycardia.
   b. Urinary retention.
   c. Diarrhea.
   d. Restlessness and agitation.

6. Mr. M. is taking levodopa (Dopar). The nurse should include the following information in her teaching:
   a. Parkinsonism symptoms will reoccur after a few years of therapy.
   b. You should always take the medication with high-protein foods.
   c. Except for a little gastrointestinal upset, you should experience no side effects from this drug.
   d. This drug will prevent the reoccurrence of symptoms for at least 5 years.

7. Which one of the following medications, if administered with levodopa-carbidopa (Sinemet), could decrease its effects?
   a. Amantadine (Symmetrel).
   b. Trihexyphenidyl (Artane).
   c. Carbidopa (Lodosyn).
   d. Bromocriptine (Parlodel).

8. Mr. P. is to be started on benztropine (Cogentin). Prior to administering this drug the nurse should assess him for
   a. diabetes mellitus.
   b. diarrhea.
   c. hypotension.
   d. tachycardia.

9. Carbidopa is administered with levodopa because
   a. it enables more levodopa to reach the brain.
   b. it decreases the side effects of levodopa.
   c. it enables levodopa to be used longer.
   d. it relieves Parkinsonism symptoms rapidly.

10. An adverse effect of _____ can result when trihexyphenidyl (Artane) is used with elderly clients.
    a. Agitation.
    b. Syncope.
    c. Confusion.
    d. Delirium.

## Critical thinking case study

Mr. P. is diagnosed with Parkinson's disease and started on benztropine (Cogentin), an anticholinergic agent.

1.  Identify the adverse effects of this medication and the nursing measures that you will use to prevent complications.

Mr. P. asks you about the progression of Parkinson's disease.

2.  Describe how you will respond to his inquiry.

Three years after initial diagnosis, the medication Mr. P. is receiving is no longer effective and the physician starts Mr. P. on levodopa-carbidopa (Sinemet).

3.  Discuss why this medication was chosen for Mr. P.

4.  Identify what you will assess for and what you will teach the client.

# CHAPTER 13

# Skeletal Muscle Relaxants

## Complete the following sentences

1. Skeletal muscle relaxants are used to _____ or _____.

2. _____ (_____) is the only muscle relaxant that acts on the muscle itself.

3. Dantrolene (Dantrium) is also indicated for prevention and treatment of _____.

4. While taking muscle relaxants, clients should be instructed not to attempt activities that require _____ or _____.

5. The drug of choice for persons with multiple sclerosis is _____ (_____).

6. Which muscle relaxants can be given IV for acute muscle spasm? _____ (_____), _____ (_____), and _____ (_____).

7. Adjunctive measures for muscle spasm include:
   a. _____.
   b. _____.
   c. _____.
   d. _____.
   e. regular exercise.

8. Muscle relaxants have not been established for safe use in _____.

9. Diazepam (Valium) should be administered at a rate of _____. This minimizes the risks of _____.

10. If methocarbamol (_____) is administered rapidly, it can cause _____, _____, and _____.

## True or false

_____ 1. Diazepam (Valium) should not be mixed in a syringe with other drugs because it is incompatible.

_____ 2. If hypersensitivity reactions occur, the dosage of the drug should be decreased.

_____ 3. Persons taking MAO inhibitors will need to increase their dose of muscle relaxants to produce the same effect.

_____ 4. Diazepam (Valium) can produce psychological or physical dependence.

_____ 5. The dosage of muscle relaxants should be increased slowly.

## Crossword puzzle

### Across

2. One of the side effects of skeletal muscle relaxants.
3. Approved for treating people with multiple sclerosis.
4. One of the several muscle relaxant drugs that should be administered with food to prevent GI distress.
6. A stroke or spinal cord injury can lead to _____.
8. The drug for prevention and treatment of malignant hyperthermia.
9. Skeletal muscle relaxants have not been proven safe for use during _____.
10. The patient should lie down while this drug is being administered via IV.

### Down

1. A nonpharmacological intervention for muscle spasm.
5. Be cautious using this drug in patients with glaucoma or cardiac arrhythmias.
7. Physically incompatible with other drugs of this class.

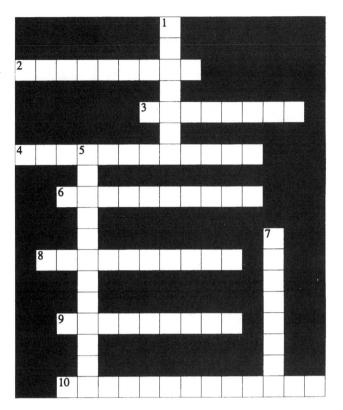

## Review questions

1. Persons taking central acting muscle relaxants should be observed for which of the following adverse effects?

   a. Hypertension.
   b. Bradycardia.
   c. Headache.
   d. Ataxia.

2. The muscle relaxant administered intravenously to treat intraoperative malignant hyperthermia is

   a. dantrolene (Dantrium).
   b. diazepam (Valium).
   c. baclofen (Lioresal).
   d. carisoprodol (Soma).

3. Which of the following disorders could be aggravated by the administration of muscle relaxants?

   a. Hypertension.
   b. Tachycardia.
   c. Diabetes mellitus.
   d. Gastrointestinal bleeding.

4. The muscle relaxant of choice for persons with multiple sclerosis is

   a. methocarbamol (Robaxin).
   b. diazepam (Valium).
   c. baclofen (Lioresal).
   d. orphenadrine citrate (Norflex).

5. This muscle relaxant can be administered parenterally for acute muscle spasm.

   a. Metaxalone (Skelaxin).
   b. Baclofen (Lioresal).
   c. Chlorzoxazone (Paraflex).
   d. Diazepam (Valium).

6. Besides administration of muscle relaxants, other measures that can help muscle spasms are

   a. weight lifting.
   b. moist heat and massage.
   c. eliminating food sources high in sodium.
   d. steroids and anti-inflammatory drugs.

7. Which of the following statements indicates that your client, who is receiving dantrolene (Dantrium), needs additional teaching?
    a. "I will not stop my medication if I experience side effects; I will contact my physician."
    b. "I should not drink alcohol while I am taking this medication."
    c. "The medicine may cause drowsiness."
    d. "The medicine will prevent the progression of my multiple sclerosis."

8. Mr. H. is started on dantrolene (Dantrium) for muscle spasticity. Which of the following lab studies should be assessed before the medication is administered?
    a. Serum glucose.
    b. Serum electrolytes.
    c. Cardiac enzymes.
    d. Liver function studies.

9. In teaching Mrs. S. about the effects of baclofen (Lioresal), the following information should be included:
    a. The medication should be taken on an empty stomach.
    b. You should expect a drop in your pulse rate.
    c. If you experience nausea, vomiting, and diarrhea, contact your physician.
    d. Skin rashes are expected and will go away in a few weeks.

10. The following muscle relaxant should be used only for short periods of time because it can produce physical and psychological addiction:
    a. Chlorzoxazone (Paraflex).
    b. Baclofen (Lioresal).
    c. Dantrolene (Dantrium).
    d. Diazepam (Valium).

## Critical thinking case study

Your client, a 28-year-old aerobics instructor, has been taking cyclobenzaprine (Flexeril) to relieve the pain associated with an ankle injury. Three weeks after her initial injury, she returns to her physician's office, still complaining of pain and requesting a prescription renewal.

1. Identify the assessment that you will do.

2. Describe your response to her request for additional medication.

3. Discuss alternatives to drug therapy.

# CHAPTER 14

# Anesthetics

## Matching exercise: terms and concepts

_____ 1. One of the most widely used anesthetics.

_____ 2. No longer used in the U.S.; still used in underdeveloped countries.

_____ 3. Given intravenously to induce anesthesia.

_____ 4. Given IM preoperatively for sedation.

_____ 5. Its effects can be reversed by neostigmine.

_____ 6. Its short duration of action makes it useful for endoscopy.

_____ 7. Used in conjunction with succinylcholine to inhibit muscle twitching.

_____ 8. Used alone for analgesia in dentistry, obstetrics, and brief surgical procedures.

_____ 9. A very potent narcotic analgesic similar to morphine whose analgesic effect lasts about 30 minutes.

_____ 10. A naturally occurring plant alkaloid that causes skeletal muscle paralysis.

_____ 11. Given to prevent excessive activity of the parasympathetic nervous system.

_____ 12. Administration of this drug preoperatively allows easier induction of anesthesia.

_____ 13. Injection of an anesthetic solution around the area to be anesthetized.

_____ 14. A solution used in spinal anesthesia that gravitates toward the head when the person is tilted in a head-down position.

_____ 15. Topical anesthetic that has a rapid onset.

A. Ether.

B. Halothane (Fluothane).

C. Midazolam (Versed).

D. Fentanyl citrate (Sublimaze).

E. Thiopental sodium (Pentothal).

F. Tubocurarine.

G. Nitrous oxide.

H. Hexafluorenium (Mylaxen)

I. Pancuronium (Pavulon).

J. Cyclopropane.

K. Succinylcholine (Anectine).

L. Glycopyrrolate (Robinul).

M. Hydroxyzine (Vistaril).

N. Field block.

O. Epidural anesthesia.

P. Hyperbaric solution.

Q. Hypobaric solution.

R. Lidocaine (Xylocaine).

## Word scramble

Unscramble the word and circle it in the word find.

1. ranthee _____
2. nafoer _____
3. neatfal _____
4. ravionn _____
5. vonpaul _____

6. niceante _____
7. neetbium _____
8. falsentu _____
9. served _____
10. verbilat _____

**Word Find**

```
B A E C C T R I S O M E T A L C H E M P N I P A N
A L T B A C I T R E M E N A R C H O R O L A C O L
C M H T R A L C O H V P E R A G A R I R I H O K C
F O R A N E R L L S S N E S S T I T H E O P H Y L
T S A N S E I O E A A A N I N N O V A R E A N I X
O C N E T I P N E L A T I E N T G E O M T R I C U
B A E A L N P A L P I T F T I O N S E C O E S N E
A N E B O N D I H E X L L G H A L A B F I N I A X
C N U C T E C H Y P A V U L O N V E R E F L E X E
K A P T A B R A P P R E M E N E I O N T A O V A N
H A H S O M T R E M O R A N G C N E J T A O C N I
A B O T P E P I R N N Q B B A T T R I P C O C T N
N C R V Q T I H T E A B I E F I A R E S T L Y H H
E N I M O R B O E H T C N X O N T S E N I M A I C
C I A N S A N T N T A I N T M E T U B I N E M N Y
T A Y N A Z I T S L A E M O R D N F S S E T T E R
O M A H V O T R A C O M M R E X N E O E I F I N T
P P T A M L R T O P A M I N E C T N L B G N O I S
A H A A D O I C N A A F N N F D D T O E V E S O I
N A T I N V E R S E D I F A E L A A M M P A L O C
T I R E E E S T L E S S N E S S U A A W I T O O M
R R F R C S E T R E O N P I I A U N U T W R I M C
Y B B L R S H N V R R S I S E N I K R E P Y H C A
X T E L B E J Q U T H Y P O A C E B R S H I S P W
A L B E L L A D O W D Y M N T E S O O T Y P A K T
```

## Review questions

1. Mrs. J. is scheduled for surgery tomorrow and she is to have an epidural anesthetic. Which of the following statements by Mrs. J. leads you to believe that she has a good understanding of the procedure?
   a. "A drug solution will be injected between my lumbar and sacral spine."
   b. "A drug solution will be injected in the area of a large nerve plexus."
   c. "I will feel nothing above or below the area anesthetized but I will be awake."
   d. "I may temporarily lose consciousness at the start of the procedure."

2. Mr. J. is agitated and "fighting" the ventilator. Which of the following medications would help maintain Mr. J. on the ventilator?
   a. Tetracaine (Pontocaine).
   b. Pancuronium (Pavulon).
   c. Thiopental sodium (Pentothal).
   d. Isoflurane (Forane).

3. Mr. J. has all of the following illnesses. For which of the following illnesses would the use of ketamine (Ketalar) be contraindicated?
   a. Hepatic failure.
   b. Diabetes.
   c. Psychosis.
   d. Renal disease.

4. Which of the following is a common complication after regional anesthesia that the nurse should be assessing for?

   a. Hypertension.

   b. Bradycardia.

   c. Urinary retention.

   d. Hypoxia.

5. Mrs. J., a 46-year-old insulin-dependent diabetic, returns to the recovery room after surgery. Her initial BP is 76/54 and her pulse is 120. What should your initial action be?

   a. Increase the rate of the IV solution.

   b. Contact her physician.

   c. Administer orange juice and sugar.

   d. Try and arouse Mrs. J. and check her BP and pulse again in 15 minutes.

6. Prior to surgery, the anesthesiologist should be made aware of any medications that will increase the effect of general anesthetic agents. These medications include

   a. anticholinergic medications.

   b. bronchodilators.

   c. diuretics.

   d. antihypertensive medications.

7. You are doing preoperative teaching with Mrs. S. Which of the following statements by Mrs. S. leads you to believe that she has understood the teaching that you have done about the adverse effects of anesthetics?

   a. "I will turn, cough, and deep breathe immediately after surgery because the temporary paralysis of respiratory muscles can lead to retained secretions."

   b. "My blood pressure will be checked regularly because they will be assessing me for hypertension."

   c. "I need to drink lots of fluids to prevent hypotension and bradycardia."

   d. "I will be drowsy for 24 hours after the surgery because of the anesthetic, so I will stay in bed."

8. Glycopyrrolate (Robinul) is administered preoperatively to prevent excessive

   a. tachycardia.

   b. bradycardia.

   c. hypertension.

   d. respiratory secretions.

9. Which of the following conditions would necessitate a larger amount of general anesthetic to be administered?

   a. Pancreatitis.

   b. Renal failure.

   c. Alcoholism.

   d. Psychosis.

10. Which of the following statements by your client leads you to believe that she understands the instructions you have given her about her preanesthetic sedation?

    a. "After I receive the medication, my family must leave and I will be immediately transported to the operating room."

    b. "I must call if I need help."

    c. "I will fall asleep and when I wake up the surgery will be over."

    d. "I can only use the bed pan."

## Critical thinking case study

Mrs. J., a 29-year-old, is admitted for a C-section. Spinal anesthesia is performed.

1. Identify two other situations in which spinal anesthesia is the preferred method.

2. Specify client behaviors that signal an adverse response to a spinal anesthetic.

3. Specify fetal responses to excessive anesthetics.

4. Discuss nursing actions that are required in the event of an adverse response.

# CHAPTER 15

# Alcohol and Other Drug Abuse

## Matching exercise: terms and concepts

_____ 1. The primary drug of abuse worldwide.

_____ 2. Symptoms of alcohol withdrawal.

_____ 3. Symptoms of amphetamine withdrawal.

_____ 4. Symptoms of barbiturate withdrawal.

_____ 5. The use of this drug results in euphoric excitement and strong psychic dependence.

_____ 6. A major danger with these drugs is their ability to impair judgment.

_____ 7. These substances are most often abused by preadolescents.

_____ 8. A potent analgesic that produces rapid, intense euphoria.

_____ 9. This drug is used as an antiemetic for clients receiving anticancer drugs.

_____ 10. A drug used in the treatment of alcohol abuse.

_____ 11. A drug used in the treatment of heroin addiction.

_____ 12. Symptoms seen with an overdose of opiate.

_____ 13. Drug administered to reverse effects of an opiate.

_____ 14. Drugs of choice for treating alcohol withdrawal.

_____ 15. Treatment of an overdose of amphetamines includes this.

A. Cocaine.

B. Alcohol.

C. Tremors, sweating, nausea, tachycardia.

D. Heroin.

E. Depression and fatigue.

F. Hallucinogenic drugs.

G. Anxiety, tremors, insomnia, weight loss.

H. Marijuana.

I. Volatile solvents (inhalants).

J. Disulfiram (Antabuse).

K. Methadone (Dolophine).

L. Naloxone (Narcan).

M. Severe respiratory depression and coma.

N. Sedation, lowering of body temperature, and administration of antipsychotic drugs.

O. Benzodiazepines

**DEFINE:**

ALCOHOLISM

PSYCHOLOGICAL DEPENDENCE

PHYSICAL DEPENDENCE

## Nursing Process

Identify four nursing diagnoses, assessment data, and nursing interventions for a person requiring drug treatment for alcoholism.

| Nursing Diagnoses | Assessment Data | Nursing Interventions |
| --- | --- | --- |
| 1. | | |
| 2. | | |
| 3. | | |
| 4. | | |

## Review questions

1. Your client is started on disulfiram (Antabuse). You know that he has a good understanding of the side effects of the medication if he states:

   a. "Antabuse can cause excessive bleeding. I'll contact my doctor if that happens."
   
   b. "The only drug that will cause a reaction when taken with Antabuse is alcohol."
   
   c. "If I ingest alcohol with Antabuse, it will cause flushing, dyspnea, and hypotension."
   
   d. "I must always take Antabuse with meals to prevent nausea and vomiting."

2. Mr. J. is admitted to the emergency room with a heroin overdose. The nurse should assess Mr. J. for

   a. seizure activity.
   
   b. respiratory depression.
   
   c. hallucinations.
   
   d. hypertension.

3. Mrs. H. is to be observed for alcohol withdrawal. Which of the following symptoms would you report to the physician?

   a. Lethargy, somnolence, vertigo.
   
   b. Diaphoresis, bradycardia, hypotension.
   
   c. Anorexia, blurred vision, headache.
   
   d. Tremors, agitation, insomnia.

4. Mr. C. is diagnosed with type II diabetes and is started on chlorpropamide (Diabinese). Which of the following statements by Mr. C. leads you to believe that he has understood the teaching that you have done?

   a. "If I drink alcohol with this medication, it may cause blurred vision."
   
   b. "If I drink alcohol, I must increase the amount of medication I am taking."
   
   c. "If I drink alcohol with this medication, it may cause my blood sugar to fluctuate."
   
   d. "If I drink alcohol, I must decrease the amount of medication I am taking."

5. Chronic alcoholism results in the malabsorption of certain vitamins and minerals. Which of the following will you need to administer to an alcoholic client?

   a. Vitamin C, vitamin D, vitamin E.
   
   b. Riboflavin, niacin, zinc.
   
   c. Thiamine, folic acid, vitamin $B_{12}$.
   
   d. Magnesium, phosphorus, vitamin $B_6$.

6. Which of the following changes commonly seen in alcoholics affects the metabolism of certain medications?

   a. Impaired carbohydrate metabolism.
   b. Increased intestinal motility.

   c. Increased production of lipids.
   d. Increased function of liver enzymes.

7. Folic acid is given to treat which of the following anemias?

   a. Sideroblastic anemia.
   b. Hemolytic anemia.

   c. Megaloblastic anemia.
   d. Iron deficiency anemia.

8. Mr. B. is admitted with an overdose of LSD. Which of the following nursing diagnoses would take priority?

   a. Ineffective individual coping related to reliance on drugs.
   b. Altered nutrition related to drug-seeking behavior.

   c. High risk for injury related to impaired judgment and impulsive behavior.
   d. Altered thought process related to drug use.

9. A drug used in the treatment of heroin addiction is

   a. naloxone (Narcan).
   b. methadone (Dolophine).

   c. disulfiram (Antabuse).
   d. chlordiazepoxide (Librium).

10. Which of the following is the best explanation why an alcoholic may require greater amounts of pain medication?

    a. There is an increased rate of metabolism of certain drugs because of enzyme induction.
    b. Increased production of lipids results in a greater distribution of fat-soluble drugs.

    c. Damage to the epithelial cells alters the absorption of certain drugs.
    d. Low albumin levels affect protein binding; therefore, smaller amounts of drugs reach their intended location.

## Critical thinking case study

M., a 28-year-old female, is admitted to your unit with symptoms of alcohol withdrawal. She was found on a park bench by the police. As a result of the admission blood work, you discover that M. is pregnant. (The learner may need additional resources to answer these questions.)

1. Describe how you will proceed with the admission history and physical of M.

2.  Discuss how M. will be treated for alcohol withdrawal.

You have observed that M. is a heavy smoker. She has now completed her treatment and is ready to go.

3.  Identify the information that you will give her prior to discharge.

4.  Discuss your discharge plan for M.

After delivery, M. decides to start disulfiram (Antabuse).

5.  Identify the information that you will provide her.

# CHAPTER 16

# Central Nervous System Stimulants

## Complete the following sentences

1. Two disorders treated with CNS stimulants are _____ and _____.

2. Narcolepsy is _____by periodic "sleep attacks."

3. Hyperkinetic syndrome occurs in _____ and is characterized by

   _____, _____, _____,

   _____, and _____.

4. Amphetamines produce _____ and _____.

   Amphetamines also increase _____and_____, produce

   _____, and slow _____. These drugs also produce

   _____.

5. Analeptic drugs stimulate _____. A major drawback is the

   adverse effect of _____.

6. Xanthine drugs increase _____ and decrease _____.

7. CNS stimulants are contraindicated in persons with _____, _____,

   _____, _____, or _____.

8. Dextroamphetamine (_____) is used to treat _____.

9. Methylphenidate (_____) is used for children with ADHD. It is usually administered
   b.i.d., Monday through Friday while children are in school. The last dose each day should be given
   _____ hours before bedtime.

10. Doxapram (_____) increases tidal volume and respiratory rate. Duration of action of a
    single dose is _____ minutes.

11. Caffeine may increase _____. It may be combined with ergot alkaloids to treat

    _____.

12. Caffeine and sodium benzoate are used as a respiratory stimulant in _____.

13. Persons taking xanthine derivatives need to limit their _____ _____ because they have
    an additive effect.

14. Children being treated for ADHD should avoid _____ in their diet.

15. Children receiving drugs for ADHD have reported suppression of _____

    and _____.

16. Adverse effects of CNS stimulants include _____, and

    _____ and _____ effects.

## Review questions

1. M., an 8-year-old with undifferentiated ADHD, is to receive methylphenidate (Ritalin) b.i.d. When are the best times to administer the drug?

   a. Before breakfast and lunch.
   b. Before breakfast and dinner.
   c. Before breakfast and h.s.
   d. Before lunch and h.s.

2. M. must be assessed for adverse effects of methylphenidate (Ritalin) which include

   a. impaired motor coordination.
   b. decreased attention span.
   c. muscle atrophy.
   d. altered growth and development.

3. After instructions about methylphenidate (Ritalin), which statement by M.'s parents would lead you to believe they need additional instruction?

   a. "M. will have warm milk, not hot chocolate, before she goes to bed."
   b. "M. can have soft drinks that don't contain caffeine."
   c. "M. can have iced tea in the summertime when the weather gets hot."
   d. "We will limit the amounts and types of candy she eats."

4. Mr. D. is diagnosed with narcolepsy and is to be started on amphetamines to treat this problem. Prior to initiating this therapy, the nurse should assess Mr. D. for the presence of the following condition that may prohibit the use of amphetamines:

   a. Diabetes mellitus.
   b. Hypertension.
   c. Asthma.
   d. Epilepsy.

5. Mr. D. should be instructed to contact the physician if he begins to experience this adverse reaction from dextroamphetamine (Dexedrine).

   a. Rash.
   b. Tachycardia.
   c. Drowsiness.
   d. Increased urinary output.

6. When clients are receiving amphetamines, they should be assessed for alteration in

   a. nutrition.
   b. urinary elimination.
   c. motor coordination.
   d. attention span.

7. Mr. H. is admitted with drug-induced CNS depression. Doxapram (Dopram) is ordered because it

   a. increases mental alertness.
   b. increases tidal volume and respiratory rate.
   c. produces bronchodilation.
   d. provides analgesia without CNS depression.

8. When doxapram (Dopram) is administered, the nurse should be assessing for the following adverse effects:

   a. Confusion.
   b. Bradycardia.
   c. Seizures.
   d. Apnea.

9. Caffeine reduces

   a. fatigue.
   b. the need for sleep.
   c. anorexia.
   d. urinary output.

10. When teaching clients about the use of caffeine, you should include the following information:

    a. It has no impact on medication that you take.
    b. It produces tolerance and habituation can occur.
    c. There are no adverse effects to ingestion of caffeine.
    d. It is effective in treating head colds.

# SECTION III

# Drugs Affecting the Autonomic Nervous System

---

## CHAPTER 17

## Physiology of the Autonomic Nervous System

### Fill in the chart

Fill in the chart below with the following terms to indicate stimulation.

Constriction
Decreases heart rate
Decreases force of contraction
Aggregation
Bronchoconstriction
Increases force of contraction

Increases heart rate
Bronchodilation
Increases motility
Decreases motility
Dilation
Glycogenolysis

#### AUTONOMIC NERVOUS SYSTEM

| PARA-SYMPATHETIC | Location | alpha$_1$ | alpha$_2$ | beta$_1$ | beta$_2$ |
|---|---|---|---|---|---|
|  | blood vessels | _____ |  |  |  |
|  | heart |  |  | _____ |  |
|  | lungs |  |  |  | _____ |
|  | GI |  |  |  | _____ |
|  | eye | _____ |  |  |  |
|  | liver |  |  |  | _____ |
|  | platelet |  | _____ |  |  |

## True or false

_____ 1. Anticholinergic drugs act by blocking the action of acetylcholine.

_____ 2. Cholinergic drugs produce bronchoconstriction.

_____ 3. Adrenergic drugs decrease myocardial contractility.

_____ 4. Adrenergic drugs may be used in the treatment of tachycardia.

_____ 5. Beta adrenergic blocking agents are given for bronchodilating effects.

_____ 6. Beta adrenergic blocking drugs may cause tachycardia.

## Review questions

1. A side effect of nonselective beta adrenergic blockers is
   a. increased heart rate.
   b. bronchoconstriction.
   c. decreased gastric motility.
   d. pupillary constriction.

2. Cholinergic drugs can produce the following side effects:
   a. Bradycardia.
   b. Trachycardia.
   c. Constipation.
   d. Increased platelet aggregation.

3. Adrenergic drugs may cause the following side effects:
   a. Bronchoconstriction.
   b. Vasodilation.
   c. Tachycardia.
   d. Diarrhea.

4. One of the physiologic effects of the release of acetylcholine is
   a. miosis.
   b. mydriasis.
   c. tachycardia.
   d. constipation.

5. Beta adrenergic blockers are used in the treatment of
   a. asthma.
   b. angina.
   c. congestive heart failure.
   d. COPD.

6. Anticholinergic drugs can produce the following side effects:
   a. Bradycardia.
   b. Tachycardia.
   c. Vasodilation.
   d. Diarrhea.

7. The use of beta adrenergic blockers is contraindicated if the client has which one of the following disorders?
   a. Peripheral vascular disease.
   b. Prostatic disease.
   c. Tachycardia.
   d. Congestive heart failure.

8. When cholinergic drugs are administered, the nurse should observe the client for which one of the following adverse effects?
   a. Vasoconstriction.
   b. Bronchoconstriction.
   c. Fluid retention.
   d. Constipation.

9. Which of the following assessments is directly related to the stimulation of the parasympathetic nervous system?
   a. Increased heart rate.
   b. Increased respiratory rate.
   c. Cold, clammy skin.
   d. Constricted pupils.

10. An expected outcome of the administration of adrenergic agents is
    a. urinary frequency.
    b. vasodilation.
    c. bronchodilation.
    d. bradycardia.

# CHAPTER 18

# Adrenergic Drugs

## Matching exercise: terms and concepts

_____ 1. A drug used to raise the blood pressure.

_____ 2. A drug that increases the force of the contraction of the heart.

_____ 3. A drug that produces bronchodilation as well as tachycardia.

_____ 4. Commonly used inhaler that produces bronchodilation.

_____ 5. A drug used for the treatment of allergic reactions, shock, and cardiac arrest.

_____ 6. A contraindication to using adrenergic agents.

_____ 7. A drug used for bronchodilation and nasal congestion; sold over the counter.

_____ 8. A substance that, when administered with adrenergic agents, has a synergistic bronchodilating effect.

_____ 9. A drug used for nasal congestion; also acts as an appetite suppressant.

_____ 10. An ophthalmic preparation that produces mydriasis but can also cause hypertension.

A. Isoproterenol (Isuprel).

B. Narrow-angle glaucoma.

C. Dopamine (Intropin).

D. Dobutamine (Dobutrex).

E. Epinephrine (Adrenalin).

F. Albuterol (Proventil).

G. Caffeine.

H. Phenylpropanolamine hydrochloride (Propagest).

I. Pseudoephedrine (Sudafed).

J. Phenylephrine (Neo-Synephrine).

## True or false

_____ 1. Epinephrine (Adrenalin) causes peripheral vasoconstriction and bronchodilation.

_____ 2. Common side effects resulting from the administration of adrenergic drugs include hypotension and bradycardia.

_____ 3. Albuterol (Proventil) should not be given to children under 12 years of age.

_____ 4. An expected outcome of the administration of Dopamine (Intropin) is increased urinary output.

_____ 5. Inhaled solutions of isoproterenol (Isuprel) may turn saliva pink.

_____ 6. When nasal decongestants are used excessively, a rebound nasal congestion can result.

_____ 7. When adrenergic agents are administered with beta blockers, the effect of the adrenergic agent is increased.

_____ 8. Epinephrine (Adrenalin) can only be administered parenterally.

_____ 9. A common side effect from the administration of epinephrine (Adrenalin) is an elevated serum glucose.

_____ 10. The usual goal of vasopressor therapy is to maintain the systolic blood pressure above 80.

## Sentence correction

Circle the word(s) that make the sentence incorrect and place the correct word(s) in the blank.

_____ 1. Ephedrine is used as a bronchodilator to treat bronchospasm.

_____ 2. An allergic reaction that produces severe respiratory distress and profound hypertension.

_____ 3. Acute asthma attacks may be precipitated by exposure to toxins.

_____ 4. Alkalosis may occur with acute bronchospasm.

_____ 5. When administering substances known to produce hypersensitivity reactions, observe the recipient carefully for 5 minutes after administration.

_____ 6. Levarterenol (Levophed) stimulates electrical and mechanical activity to produce myocardial contraction.

_____ 7. Ephedrine is used to treat Marfan's syndrome, a sudden attack of unconsciousness brought on by heart block.

_____ 8. Pseudoephedrine is an ingredient in cold medications.

_____ 9. Isoproterenol (Isuprel) may cause chest pain and bradycardia.

_____ 10. Terbutaline (Brethine) is not recommended for children over the age of 12.

_____ 11. When giving dopamine (Intropin), observe for improved breathing.

_____ 12. When excessive amounts of nasal decongestants are used, hypertension can result.

_____ 13. When assessing for the effectiveness of vasopressors, you should assess blood pressures and the person's respiratory status.

_____ 14. Anticholinergic drugs decrease the effects of adrenergic drugs.

_____ 15. Metaraminol (Aramine) is used for bronchodilation and vasoconstriction.

## Review questions

1. The use of isoproterenol (Isuprel) is contraindicated in persons with the following conditions:
   a. Diabetes mellitus.
   b. Tachycardia.
   c. Hypotension.
   d. Bronchoconstriction.

2. An expected outcome after the administration of a vasopressor is
   a. increased urinary output.
   b. headache.
   c. flushing of the head and neck.
   d. rapid respirations.

3. The drug of choice for treating shock due to an anaphylactic reaction is
   a. isoproterenol (Isuprel).
   b. dopamine (Intropin).
   c. dobutamine (Dobutrex).
   d. epinephrine (Adrenalin).

4. Adrenergic drugs are contraindicated in which of the following conditions?
   a. Congestive heart failure.
   b. Asthma.
   c. Narrow-angle glaucoma.
   d. Diabetes mellitus.

5. Prolonged use of high doses of dopamine (Intropin), a vasopressor, may result in
   a. myocardial infarction secondary to arterial embolization.
   b. angina secondary to vasospasm.
   c. seizures secondary to diminished blood supply to the brain.
   d. gangrene secondary to peripheral vasoconstriction.

6. The most common route for administering epinephrine (Adrenalin) is
   a. oral.
   b. intramuscular.
   c. intravenous.
   d. subcutaneous.

7. Which of the following comments by Mr. J.'s wife leads you to believe that she has a good understanding of why her husband is receiving dobutamine (Dubutrex)? The doctor ordered the medication to:
   a. "Increase the force of the contraction of my husband's heart."
   b. "Increase my husband's heart rate."
   c. "Improve his peripheral circulation."
   d. "Decrease his blood pressure."

8. Mr. J. was given epinephrine (Adrenalin) for hypotension and bradycardia. The physician now orders isoproterenol (Isuprel). What will you do?
   a. Refuse to give the medication.
   b. Administer the medication as ordered.
   c. Schedule the medication for 4 hours after the administration of the Adrenalin.
   d. Give only a portion of the dose and observe for side effects; if no side effects occur, give the remainder of the dose.

9. After a breathing treatment with isoproterenol (Isuprel), your client calls you into the room to show you her sputum and states,"I'm getting worse. Look, I have blood in my sputum." Your best response would be:
   a. "The pink color is due to the irritation in your throat caused by coughing."
   b. "I will contact your physician and send a sputum specimen."
   c. "It is common to see pink sputum when isoproterenol (Isuprel) is given by inhalation."
   d. "You have no need to be alarmed. This is a common side effect."

10. Which of the following medications, if administered concurrently with adrenergic drugs, will increase their effect?
    a. Beta adrenergic blockers.
    b. Xanthines.
    c. Thiazide diuretics.
    d. Antipsychotics.

## Critical thinking case study

Mr. J. has a myocardial infarction and develops right-sided heart failure. The physician orders an IV drip of dopamine (Intropin). (The learner may need to use additional sources to answer these questions.)

1. Explain why this drug was ordered.

2.  Identify what nursing assessments you will be performing and your rationale for each.

Mr. J.'s condition begins to deteriorate. The physician adds dobutamine (Dubutrex) to the medical regime.

3.  Explain why this drug was added to the medical regime and what the expected therapeutic effect is.

Mr. J.'s heart rate drops to 40 and the physician orders epinephrine (Adrenalin).

4.  Identify the side effects of this medication that you will be assessing for.

# CHAPTER 19

# Antiadrenergic Drugs

## Matching exercise: terms and concepts

_____ 1. Used for the treatment of supraventricular tachycardia.

_____ 2. This drug is valuable in the treatment of glaucoma.

_____ 3. The drug of choice for treating hypertensive emergencies.

_____ 4. Clients use this drug to prevent migraine headaches.

_____ 5. A selective beta blocker used to treat a myocardial infarction.

_____ 6. When nonselective beta blockers are administered, this can result.

_____ 7. This drug is effective in treating ventricular arrhythmias.

_____ 8. When this drug is administered with beta blockers, heart block can result.

_____ 9. This can be administered with beta blockers for treatment of unresponsive hypertension.

_____ 10. When this drug is administered concurrently with beta adrenergic blockers, it will decrease the effect of the beta adrenergic blocking agent.

A. Labetalol (Trandate).

B. Atenolol (Tenormin).

C. Difficulty in breathing.

D. Propranolol (Inderal).

E. Esmolol (Brevibloc).

F. Betaxolol (Betoptic).

G. Digoxin (Lanoxin).

H. Prazosin (Minipress).

I. Acebutolol (Sectral).

J. Isoproterenol (Isuprel).

K. Blurred vision.

## True or false

_____ 1. Atenolol (Tenormin) or nadolol (Corgard) is the drug of choice for persons with hepatic failure because they are eliminated by the kidney.

_____ 2. The use of beta adrenergic blockers is contraindicated in children.

_____ 3. When persons ingest alcohol, adverse effects of alpha adrenergic blocking agents can reappear.

_____ 4. If bradycardia occurs as a result of the administration of beta adrenergic blockers, atropine can be given to increase the heart rate.

_____ 5. Pindolol (Visken), acebutolol (Sectral), carteolol (Cartrol), and penbutolol (Levatol) are more likely to cause bradycardia than other beta adrenergic blocking agents.

## Beta Receptor Sites

Beta adrenergic blocking agents vie with epinephrine and norepinephrine for available receptor sites on cell membranes. Figure 19-1 illustrates the release of these naturally occurring catecholamines that are shown surrounding the nerve ending and competing with a beta adrenergic blocking drug to occupy receptor sites on the cell surface.

### PART A

Label the parts of Figure 19-1 using terms from the following list.

Epinephrine and norepinephrine    Myocardial or other cell tissue
Beta adrenergic blocking drug     Nerve endings
Receptor site

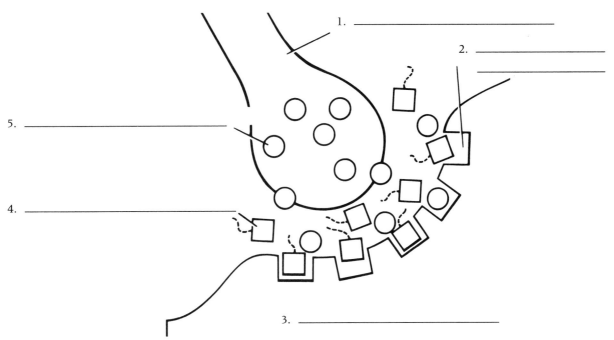

1. _____

2. _____
   _____

3. _____

4. _____

5. _____

**FIGURE 19-1**

### PART B

Using this receptor site competition theory, explain why beta adrenergic blocking agents, such as propranolol (Inderal), are used to overcome the effects of epinephrine and norepinephrine in the treatment of hypertension, arrhythmias, angina pectoris, and myocardial infarction.

## Sentence correction

Circle the word(s) that make the sentence incorrect. Place the correct word(s) in the space provided.

_____ 1. Nadolol (Corgard) is the oldest beta blocking agent.

_____ 2. Acebutolol (Sectral) is a nonselective beta blocker used to treat hypertension.

_____ 3. Esmolol (Brevibloc) is the drug of choice to treat hypertension.

_____ 4. A nonselective beta blocker used to treat glaucoma is pindolol (Visken).

_____ 5. The beta blocker of choice for treating migraine headaches is levobunolol (Betagan).

_____ 6. Metoprolol (Lopressor) is an alpha blocker used for the treatment of hypertensive emergencies.

_____ 7. A cardioselective beta blocker used for the treatment of angina is penbutolol (Levatol).

_____ 8. Selective beta blockers should not be used for persons with respiratory diseases.

_____ 9. A nonselective beta blocker used for the treatment of a myocardial infarction is levobunolol (Betagan).

_____ 10. Beta adrenergic blocking agents are contraindicated when the individual has had a stroke.

_____ 11. Timolol (Timoptic) reduces intraocular pressure by increasing the formation of aqueous humor.

_____ 12. The term _selective_ indicates that those drugs have more effect on beta$_2$ receptors.

_____ 13. Beta blockers are likely to cause tachycardia.

_____ 14. Beta blockers that are highly water soluble are more likely to cause depression, nightmares, insomnia, and hallucinations.

_____ 15. In the presence of hepatic disease, the dosage of timolol (Blocadren) should be increased.

## Review questions

1. Which of the following behaviors by Mr. B. who is receiving atenolol (Tenormin) for hypertension indicates successful teaching?
   a. Using ibuprofen (Motrin) instead of aspirin.
   b. Drinking 8 glasses of water daily.
   c. Eating foods high on roughage.
   d. Taking pulse rate daily.

2. Mr. P. has hypertension and angina. Which of the following beta adrenergic blocking agents would be most effective for treating Mr. P.?
   a. Acebutolol (Sectral).
   b. Atenolol (Tenormin).
   c. Esmolol (Brevibloc).
   d. Metoprolol (Lopressor).

3. Which of the following beta adrenergic blocking agents would be most effective in treating migraine headaches?
   a. Propranolol (Inderal).
   b. Nadolol (Corgard).
   c. Timolol (Blocadren).
   d. Acebutolol (Sectral).

4. An expected outcome of the administration of beta adrenergic blocking agents is
   a. increased glucose production.
   b. decreased cardiac perfusion.
   c. decreased cardiac output.
   d. increased oxygen consumption.

5. Mr. C. is receiving acebutolol (Sectral) for multifocal premature testicular contractions. It is important to assess Mr. C.'s pulse rate as well as his

   a. breath sounds.
   b. blood pressure.

   c. blood sugar.
   d. orientation.

6. Which of the following statements by Mrs. H. leads you to believe that she understands the teaching that you have done regarding nadolol (Corgard)?

   a. "If I experience side effects, I will not stop taking the medication."
   b. "I am not allowed to have any caffeine."

   c. "Smoking will not reduce the effectiveness of the medication."
   d. "I must have my blood pressure taken daily."

7. The following drug, when administered with propranolol (Inderal), will increase the effect of Inderal:

   a. Atropine.
   b. Digoxin (Lanoxin).

   c. Isoproterenol (Isuprel).
   d. Levarterenol (Levophed).

8. Which of the following instructions should be included when you are discharging a client on metoprolol (Lopressor)?

   a. The drug should only be taken before bedtime.
   b. Report weight loss of more than 2 lbs. in 1 week.

   c. Take the medication on an empty stomach to enhance its absorption.
   d. Weakness and dizziness are common but usually disappear with continued use.

9. Mr. P. is taking propranolol (Inderal). Which of the following symptoms related to beta adrenergic blockers should be reported immediately?

   a. A pulse rate of 58.
   b. Ankle edema.

   c. Nausea and anorexia.
   d. Bruising.

10. In reviewing Mr. J.'s history, you discover that he has a history of depression, myocardial infarction, peripheral vascular disease, and thyrotoxicosis. Which one of these diagnoses would you discuss with the physician before administering a beta adrenergic blocker?

   a. Myocardial infarction.
   b. Peripheral vascular disease.

   c. Depression.
   d. Thyrotoxicosis.

## Critical thinking case study

Miss C., a 22-year-old college senior, is diagnosed with hyperthyroidism and started on propranolol (Inderal) for treatment of tachycardia.

1. Prior to initiating the treatment, what assessments will you do?

2. Identify the specific instructions you will give her regarding the medication.

A decision is made to perform a thyroidectomy. Two weeks before surgery, Miss C. arrives at the office, complaining of nausea and vomiting and she wonders if she should continue the medication.

3. Identify the subjective and objective assessments you will perform and your rationale.

4. Describe how you will address Miss C.'s concerns and what teaching you will do to prepare her for the surgery.

# CHAPTER 20

# Cholinergic Drugs

## Complete the following sentences

1. Cholinergic drugs stimulate the _____ nervous system.

2. Direct-acting cholinergic drugs cause

   a. _____ heart rate.

   b. _____ contractility of gastrointestinal smooth muscle.

   c. _____ sphincters.

   d. _____ contractility of smooth muscle of the bladder.

   e. _____ contractility of bronchial smooth muscle.

   f. _____ respiratory secretions.

   g. _____ pupils.

## Match the drug with its action

_____ 1. Bethanechol (Urecholine).

_____ 2. Neostigmine (Prostigmin).

_____ 3. Edrophonium (Tensilon).

_____ 4. Ambenonium (Mytelase).

_____ 5. Physostigmine salicylate (Antilirium).

A. Used as an antidote for tubocurarine and other skeletal muscle relaxants.

B. Used to diagnose myasthenia gravis.

C. Used to treat myasthenia gravis.

D. Used for urinary retention, gastric atony, paralytic ileus, and gastroesophageal reflux.

E. Used as an antidote for "atropine poisoning."

## True or false

_____ 1. The dosage of anticholinesterase drugs may need to be increased if a client develops an infection.

_____ 2. Bethanechol (Urecholine) should be administered with meals.

_____ 3. Hypertension is a common side effect of cholinergic drugs.

_____ 4. When antihistamines are administered concurrently with cholinergic drugs, they decrease the effect of the cholinergic drug.

_____ 5. Pyridostigmine (Mestinon) is taken at bedtime to prevent the client from experiencing an inability to swallow upon awakening.

## Review questions

1. Your client, who has been receiving ambenonium (Mytelase) for 1 week, develops respiratory difficulty 1 hour after you administer the medication. As you think through possible explanations for the appearance of this symptom, you determine that your client may be experiencing
   a. myasthenic crisis.
   b. cholinergic crisis.
   c. anaphylactic reaction.
   d. pulmonary edema.

2. Pyridostigmine (Mestinon) is to be administered three times a day. Which is the recommended schedule for administration of this drug?
   a. 9 A.M., 1 P.M., 5 P.M.
   b. 10 A.M., 2 P.M., 6 P.M.
   c. 8 A.M., 4 P.M., 12 P.M.
   d. 10 A.M., 4 P.M., 10 P.M.

3. You will know that ambenonium (Mytelase) has been beneficial for your client with myasthenia gravis if the client exhibits the following within hours after the administration of the drug:
   a. Movement of the eyelids.
   b. Decreased adventitious breath sounds.
   c. Decreased muscle spasms.
   d. Increased urinary output.

4. After receiving bethanechol (Urecholine), Mr. G.'s pulse drops from 80 to 70. You should
   a. contact the physician immediately.
   b. know that a drop in pulse rate is common with this drug.
   c. check his pulse every hour for the next 24 hours.
   d. have Mr. G. walk in the hall for 30 minutes, then recheck his pulse.

5. Mr. J. is receiving a cholinergic agent and his pulse drops to 50. The treatment of choice for bradycardia is to administer
   a. anticholinergic drugs.
   b. antihistamines.
   c. adrenergic blocking agents.
   d. cardiotonics.

6. When administering cholinergic drugs, the nurse should assess the client for toxic effects of the drugs which include
   a. paralytic ileus.
   b. abdominal distension.
   c. hypertension.
   d. muscle weakness.

7. The nurse knows that the client has understood her teaching about bethanechol (Urecholine) if he states:
   a. "I will take the medicine before meals."
   b. "I must drink plenty of fluids to prevent constipation."
   c. "I must eat six small meals a day."
   d. "I will take a stool softener with the Urecholine."

8. You are admitting Mr. B. to the unit. The physician has ordered neostigmine (Prostigmin) for urinary retention. Which of the diseases in Mr. B.'s past medical history should you make the physician aware of before administering the medication?
   a. Diabetes mellitus.
   b. Hypertension.
   c. Asthma.
   d. Migraine headaches.

9. Mrs. P., with myasthenia gravis, is to receive pyridostigmine (Mestinon) at bedtime. Mrs. P. asks you why she must take the medication at bedtime. Your best reply is:
   a. "You will have fewer side effects if you take the drug this way."
   b. "By taking the medicine at night, it minimizes your secretions in the morning."
   c. "By taking the drug at night, skin rashes are less likely to occur."
   d. "If you take the drug at bedtime, you will be better able to swallow when you awaken."

10. Which of the following cholinergic drugs is the drug of choice for "atropine poisoning"?
    a. Bethanechol (Urecholine).
    b. Neostigmine (Prostigmin).
    c. Edrophonium (Tensilon).
    d. Physostigmine salicylate (Antilirium).

## Critical thinking case study

J., a 9-year-old weighing 66 lbs., is admitted to your unit following surgery for a ruptured appendix. He has an nasogastric tube to intermittent suction and a Foley catheter in place. No bowel sounds are auscultated upon his return. (The learner may need to use additional sources to answer the questions below.)

1. Discuss why it is common for there to be no bowel sounds after abdominal surgery and when you can expect bowel sounds to return.

Three days after surgery, J.'s abdomen is distended, he has only faint hypoactive bowel sounds, and he is having difficulty in voiding. The physician orders bethanechol (Urecholine) 5 mg t.i.d.

2. Identify why the physician ordered this medication and whether the dose the physician ordered is within the therapeutic range for J.

3. Identify what you will expect to see.

You perform your morning assessment and find that J.'s pupils are constricted. His pulse is 110, respirations 16, blood pressure 80/60, and temperature 102°F. J. complains of a headache and nausea. You notice that his bed is wet from perspiration and he has a rash.

4.  Identify which signs/symptoms from your assessment are directly related to the cholinergic drug he is taking and what your nursing actions will be.

After the fourth dose of bethanechol (Urecholine), J. becomes short of breath.

5.  Identify and prioritize your nursing actions.

# CHAPTER 21

# Anticholinergic Drugs

## Complete the following sentences

1. Anticholinergic drugs block the action of _____ on the _____ nervous system.

2. The effects that anticholinergic drugs have on the body include:

   a. _____

   b. _____

   c. _____

   d. _____

   e. _____

   f. _____

   _____

   _____

   _____

3. GI disorders in which anticholinergics are useful include: _____,

   _____, _____, _____, _____, and

   _____.

4. Anticholinergics are used in ophthalmology to aid in _____ or _____ because

   they produce _____ effects.

5. Atropine is given to _____ the heart rate.

6. When a client is experiencing bronchoconstriction, ipratropium (Atrovent) may be given by

   _____.

7. Anticholinergic drugs are used with clients who have enuresis, paraplegia, or neurogenic bladder

   to _____.

8. Atropine and glycopyrrolate (Robinul) are used preoperatively to reduce _____

   and to prevent _____.

9. Conditions that would be aggravated by the use of anticholinergic drugs include:

   _____, _____, _____,

   _____, and _____ unless bradycardia is present.

10. Atropine is the _____ of anticholinergic drugs and can be administered _____, _____, _____, _____, _____, and by _____.

11. Hyoscyamine (Anaspaz) is a belladonna alkaloid used for gastrointestinal and urinary tract disorders that cause _____, _____, and _____.

12. Scopolamine is also used for _____. It can be administered as a _____ and it is effective for _____ hrs.

13. _____ (Artane) is used for initial treatment of _____. It is also effective in treating _____ caused by antipsychotic drugs.

14. _____ (Cogentin) is used for prevention and treatment of _____.

15. Flavoxate (Urispas) relieves _____, _____, _____, and _____.

16. Oxybutynin (_____) increases _____ and decreases _____.

17. Common adverse reactions from anticholinergic drugs that the elderly experience include: _____, _____, _____, _____, _____, _____, and _____.

## True or false

_____  1. Meperidine (Demerol) and atropine cannot be mixed in the same syringe.

_____  2. Saunas should be avoided by persons taking anticholinergic drugs.

_____  3. Anticholinergic drugs are used to produce pupillary constriction.

_____  4. Persons taking anticholinergics for peptic ulcer disease should also drink large amounts of milk to decrease gastric acid secretion.

_____  5. Dental caries and loss of teeth can occur from decreased saliva production due to administration of anticholinergic drugs.

## Matching exercise

Match the generic and trade names of the anticholinergic drugs.

_____  1. Urispas.

_____  2. Cogentin.

_____  3. Robinul.

_____  4. Anaspaz.

_____  5. Ditropan.

A. Glycopyrrolate.

B. Hyoscyamine.

C. Flavoxate.

D. Benztropine.

E. Oxybutynin.

## Review questions

1. The physician has ordered a scopolamine patch for motion sickness for Mrs. Z. Which statement by Mrs. Z. leads you to believe she knows how to use the patch?

   a. "I will place it on my chest each morning after I shower."

   b. "I will use it only if I feel sick to my stomach."

   c. "I will change the patch every 4 hours."

   d. "I will change the patch every 3 days."

2. Which of the following drugs is used for initial treatment of Parkinsonism?

   a. Flavoxate (Urispas).

   b. Benztropine (Cogentin).

   c. Trihexyphenidyl (Artane).

   d. Oxybutynin (Ditropan).

3. Mr. S. is taking propantheline bromate (Pro-Banthine) for peptic ulcer disease. Which of the following measures would also decrease gastric secretion?

   a. Drinking large amounts of milk throughout the day.

   b. Eating a snack before bedtime.

   c. Eliminating caffeine-containing beverages from his diet.

   d. Avoiding fatty foods.

4. The physician orders a preoperative medication glycopyrrolate (Robinul) 0.1 mg and meperidine (Demerol) 50 mg IM. Before administering these medications, you should assess your client for the following disorder:

   a. Tachycardia.

   b. Glaucoma.

   c. Hypertension.

   d. Diabetes mellitus.

5. After surgery, Mrs. A., who received glycopyrrolate (Robinul) and meperidine (Demerol) preoperatively, complains of mouth dryness. A teaching response to her would be:

   a. "This is caused by your preoperative medication which decreased your salivation. It is only temporary and will improve."

   b. "This is caused by loss of body fluid which is induced by glycopyrrolate (Robinul)."

   c. "You are probably dehydrated. The IV fluids you are receiving will correct the problem."

   d. "Do not worry about it; the dryness will go away."

6. Atropine is prescribed to treat

   a. blurred vision.

   b. bradycardia.

   c. paralytic ileus.

   d. urinary retention.

7. Persons taking anticholinergic medications should be instructed to eat foods that are

   a. high in protein.

   b. low in fat.

   c. high in fiber.

   d. low in sodium.

8. Anticholinergics

   a. inhibit gastric motility and secretions.

   b. stimulate the release of acetylcholine.

   c. increase respiratory tract secretions.

   d. increase secretion of sweat glands.

9. Anticholinergic drugs are given to paraplegics to

   a. increase peristalsis.

   b. increase bladder capacity.

   c. prevent vagal stimulation.

   d. reduce respiratory secretions.

10. Mr. J., age 75, is started on flavoxate (Urispas) to relieve dysuria and urgency. One of the adverse effects of anticholinergics that he should be made aware of includes

    a. skin rash.

    b. headache.

    c. weight gain.

    d. blurred vision.

## Critical thinking case study

Mr. P., a 76-year-old man, is brought to the hospital because he fainted at home. He is alert and oriented but weak. When you check Mr. P.'s apical pulse, you find it to be 40. The physician diagnoses heart block and administers atropine. Soon after the administration of atropine, Mr. P. becomes agitated and confused. (The learner may need to use additional sources to answer the questions below.)

1.  Identify and prioritize your nursing actions.

Mr. P. is again oriented and complains of dry mouth and blurred vision.

2.  Describe your response to Mr. P.

3.  Identify and prioritize your nursing actions.

# Drugs Affecting the Endocrine System

---

CHAPTER **22**

## Physiology of the Endocrine System

---

## Matching exercise: terms and concepts

____ 1. Helps maintain fluid balance.

____ 2. Influences carbohydrate storage.

____ 3. Promotes sodium retention and potassium loss.

____ 4. The adrenal medulla secretes this hormone.

____ 5. These hormones regulate the metabolic rate of the body.

____ 6. This hormone regulates calcium and phosphate metabolism.

____ 7. Regulates the metabolism of glucose, lipids, and proteins.

____ 8. Promotes the development of secondary sex characteristics in females.

____ 9. Regulates the development of male characteristics.

____ 10. Helps prepare the mammary glands for lactation.

A. Parathyroid hormone.

B. Glucagon.

C. Testicular hormone.

D. ADH.

E. Glucocorticoids.

F. Mineralocorticoid.

G. Estrogen.

H. Progesterone.

I. Epinephrine.

J. Thyroid hormones.

## True or false

_____ 1. The length of the physiological effects of endocrine hormone varies from minutes to hours.

_____ 2. All hormones are secreted by the pituitary gland.

_____ 3. Cancerous tumors can produce hormones.

_____ 4. Steroid hormones are synthesized from amino acids.

_____ 5. Secretion of all pituitary hormones is controlled by the hypothalamus.

## Review questions

1. Insulin
   a. stimulates the growth of cells, bones, and muscles.
   b. raises blood glucose levels by promoting hepatic glycogenolysis.
   c. is necessary for growth and development in children.
   d. regulates osmolality of extracellular fluids.

2. When an individual is placed in a stressful situation, increased amounts of the following hormone will be excreted:
   a. Epinephrine.
   b. Insulin.
   c. Estrogen.
   d. Thyroxine.

3. Mrs. J. is admitted with elevated blood sugar, weakness and irritability. Based on Mrs. J.'s symptoms, the nurse would suspect an abnormality in which of the following endocrine glands?
   a. Adrenal.
   b. Thyroid.
   c. Pancreas.
   d. Parathyroid.

4. M. A., a 6-year-old, is diagnosed with hypothyroidism. Her physician prescribes thyroid hormone replacement because an adequate thyroid level is necessary for
   a. regulation of metabolism and growth and development.
   b. regulation of calcium and phosphate metabolism.
   c. development of most secondary sexual characteristics.
   d. regulation of sodium and potassium balance.

5. Antidiuretic hormone is secreted by the body to control
   a. blood volume
   b. serum glucose levels.
   c. osmolarity of body fluids.
   d. serum calcium levels.

6. Glucocorticoids influence
   a. the promotion of potassium retention and sodium loss.
   b. metabolism of glucose, lipids, and proteins.
   c. the development of feminine characteristics.
   d. carbohydrate storage and protein catabolism.

7. The gastrointestinal mucosa secretes which of the following hormones that is important in the digestive process?
   a. Liothyronine.
   b. Cholecystokinin.
   c. Tetraiodothyronine.
   d. Prolactin.

8. This hormone is normally produced by the kidneys to stimulate the bone marrow to produce red blood cells. A synthetic hormone has been developed for persons in end-stage renal failure to mimic the hormone below:
   a. Gastrin.
   b. Enterogastrone.
   c. Erythropoietin.
   d. Secretin.

9. Adrenal corticosteroids are administered for the treatment of
   a. Addison's disease.
   b. Cushing's disease.
   c. Marfan's syndrome.
   d. Parkinson's disease.

10. Mr. P. is an insulin-dependent diabetic who is started on Synthroid. The addition of Synthroid
    a. will have no effect on his insulin requirements.
    b. may increase his insulin requirements.
    c. may decrease his insulin requirements.
    d. is likely to cause a toxic effect that must be carefully assessed.

# CHAPTER 23

# Hypothalamic and Pituitary Hormones

## Matching exercise: terms and concepts

_____ 1. Stimulates the adrenal cortex to produce adreno-corticosteroid.

_____ 2. Regulates secretion of thyroid hormones.

_____ 3. Stimulates functions of sex glands.

_____ 4. Stimulates hormone production by the gonads of both sexes.

_____ 5. Plays a part in milk production in nursing mothers.

_____ 6. Causes reabsorption of water.

_____ 7. Excessive production of this hormone can result in giantism.

_____ 8. The most widely used drug for diabetes insipidus.

_____ 9. Drug used to induce labor.

_____ 10. Drug used in the treatment of infertility to induce ovulation.

_____ 11. Drug used as a diagnostic test in suspected adrenal insufficiency.

_____ 12. Sudden discontinuation of this drug may cause weakness, fatigue, and hypotension.

_____ 13. Prolonged administration of this drug can cause edema and breast enlargement.

_____ 14. Adverse effects of this drug include headache, nasal congestion, nausea, and hyponatremia.

_____ 15. This drug given concurrently with vasopressin will increase its effect.

A. Follicle-stimulating hormone.

B. Oxytocin (Pitocin).

C. Menotropins (Pergonal).

D. Luteinizing hormone.

E. Cosyntropin (Cortrosyn).

F. Human chorionic gonadotropin.

G. Thyrotropin-releasing hormone.

H. Vasopressin (Pitressin).

I. Antidiuretic hormone (ADH).

J. Prolactin.

K. Corticotropin (ACTH).

L. Desmopressin acetate (Stimate).

M. Corticotropin.

N. Growth hormone.

O. Trimethaphen (Arfonad).

## Review questions

1. Your client is admitted with a diagnosis of diabetes insipidus. Lypressin is ordered. The advantage of this medication over others used for diabetes insipidus is that it can be administered

   a. orally.

   b. rectally.

   c. intranasally.

   d. parenterally.

2. Nursing actions for children receiving growth hormones should include

   a. record height and weight daily.

   b. periodic x-rays to determine bone growth.

   c. record blood pressures weekly.

   d. monitoring of serum glucose levels.

3. You know that your client who is being treated for diabetes insipidus understands the teaching that you have done regarding Lypressin if she states the following:

   a. "My intake and output should be approximately equal."

   b. "My urine specific gravity should be 1.005."

   c. "I will weigh myself weekly and report a weight gain of more than 2 lbs."

   d. "I will only eat foods low in sodium."

4. Mrs. G.'s labor is not progressing so her physician starts an IV drip of oxytocin (Pitocin). The nurse should be observing Mrs. G. for

   a. hypertension.

   b. respiratory distress.

   c. uterine rupture.

   d. confusion.

5. Which of the following medications, if administered with vasopressin, would increase its effect?

   a. Estrogen.

   b. Calcium.

   c. Cosyntropin (Cortrosyn).

   d. Chlorpropamide (Diabinese).

6. Your client is receiving corticotropin (ACTH). Which of the following instructions should be received before he goes home?

   a. Weigh yourself daily.

   b. Do not eat foods high in vitamin C.

   c. Have your blood pressure checked weekly.

   d. Do not stop the medication abruptly.

7. Persons taking corticotropin (ACTH) may develop

   a. hypokalemia.

   b. hypoglycemia.

   c. hyponatremia.

   d. a rash.

8. Adverse affects that the nurse administering vasopressin should assess for include

   a. chest pain.

   b. arrhythmias.

   c. hypotension.

   d. rash.

9. Desmopressin (Stimate) can cause hyponatremia. Symptoms that the nurse should be observing for include

   a. confusion.

   b. bradycardia.

   c. blurred vision.

   d. pleural effusion.

10. Your client is taking menotropins (Pergonal). Which of the following statements by your client leads you to believe that she has a good understanding of the side effects of this drug?

    a. "If I get pregnant, I know that I am at a higher risk for miscarriage because of this drug."

    b. "I will watch for bleeding because I know uterine rupture can occur."

    c. "This medication can elevate my blood pressure so I will have it checked regularly."

    d. "I may have twins as a result of taking this drug."

## Critical thinking case study

Ms. G., an 18-year-old prima 1 gravida 0, has been in labor for 6 hours and her labor is not progressing. Her physician decides to start an oxytocin (Pitocin) drip.

1.  Explain to Ms. G. the rationale for starting this medication and what she can expect.

The order for the oxytocin (Pitocin) reads: 1–2 milliunits/min; increase by 1–2 milliunits every 15 minutes.

2.  Discuss why the medication is administered this way.

One hour after starting the oxytocin (Pitocin) Ms. G. starts screaming, "I can't take the pain; do something."

3.  Identify and prioritize your nursing actions.

Ms. G. delivers an 8 lb., 8 oz healthy baby boy. After delivery, the physician wants the oxytocin (Pitocin) drip continued. Ms. G. starts crying and says,"Why can't they stop the medication now that I've had the baby?"

4.  Identify your best response.

# CHAPTER 24

# Corticosteroids

## True or false

_____ 1. Secretion of corticosteroids normally decreases during periods of stress.

_____ 2. Secretion of corticosteroids is normally controlled by a positive feedback mechanism.

_____ 3. Endogenous corticosteroids are those obtained from a source outside the human body.

_____ 4. Glucocorticoids may cause delayed wound healing and tissue wasting as a result of protein depletion.

_____ 5. Glucocorticoids may cause hyperglycemia and diabetes mellitus as a result of increased production and decreased use of glucose.

_____ 6. Glucocorticoids are often given therapeutically for anti-inflammatory effects.

_____ 7. Aldosterone conserves water and sodium and eliminates potassium.

_____ 8. Sex hormones are produced by the adrenal glands of both men and women.

_____ 9. Corticosteroid drugs cure the diseases for which they are given.

_____ 10. A major adverse effect of corticosteroid drug therapy is suppression of the HPA axis.

_____ 11. Glucocorticoid drugs have about the same anti-inflammatory effects when given in equivalent doses.

_____ 12. Long-term corticosteroid drug therapy should be reserved for life-threatening conditions or severe, disabling symptoms that do not respond to other measures.

_____ 13. For people on corticosteroid therapy, dosage must be tapered slowly when the drug is discontinued.

_____ 14. Alternate day therapy is used for children receiving corticosteroids because it does not affect their growth.

_____ 15. When corticosteroids are being used for adrenal insufficiency, they should be administered between 6 P.M. and 9 P.M.

## Undesirable effects of drug administration

Place a checkmark by the following words or phrases that indicate adverse effects of corticosteroid drug therapy.

_____ 1. Dehydration.

_____ 2. Rounded or "moon" face.

_____ 3. Hyperglycemia.

_____ 4. Delayed wound healing.

_____ 5. Edema.

_____ 6. Inhibition of bone growth.

_____ 7. Oliguria.

_____ 8. Hypokalemia.

_____ 9. Hypertension.

_____ 10. Tissue wasting.

_____ 11. Impaired ability to cope with stress.

_____ 12. Euphoria.

_____ 13. Cushing's disease.

_____ 14. Hypernatremia.

_____ 15. Hypercorticism.

_____ 16. Nausea and vomiting.

_____ 17. Change in sleep patterns.

_____ 18. Diarrhea.

_____ 19. Excessive sweating.

_____ 20. Depression.

_____ 21. Acne.

_____ 22. Increased intraocular pressure.

_____ 23. Anorexia.

_____ 24. Peptic ulcer disease.

## Word scramble

Provide the trade name for each generic name, then circle the trade name in the word find.

1. beclomethasone _____

2. betamethasone _____

3. fludrocortisone _____

4 flunisolide _____

5. triamcinolone
   hexacetonide _____

6. hydrocortisone _____

7. methylprednisolone _____

8. prednisolone _____

9. cortisone _____

10. dexamethasone _____

11. paramethasone _____

12. triamcinolone _____

13. prednisolone
    sodium phosphate _____

14. prednisone _____

**Word Find**

```
A P P L H E X N O T H S B H Y P O F T I L C L C E
B F G H D J K A D R E N E R G I C E N B E C T A Z
C O L A E N E C M R A I S S A N L L X Q K O V Z S
D E A N L V C D N C H T N H X Y Z T I P L R D N E
E G G H T D R O E O N I R Y L A R N V R H T L P O
F O N T A D I L N C A Y Y D O D A V P P J O F N V
A N L E S C B R E I K X F E H T G N A E B N O S B
R I F L O R I N E F L U A L A C A A I D A E U K L
O E E U N R E T O R P M X T T O S H R F R N O H A
Y P X C E L E S T O N E D R K B B L K A O T L R N
A J R E C L N O N O T D H A R I S T O C O R T S B
H Y P O F T I L C L C R E S F G H H J N K K A D R
E N E R G I C E L N B O E O T D A Z O L O L A N E
C M R A I S S I A N E L L L X E K V Z S X C W C A
H L P O D I R L A U D I D N A C A Y Y O D A U P J
R I L U A E A C A A I D A V H A L D R O N E H A P
D K B E C L A O T L R N A Y J D R E C L N O S T Y
M P E N A M B E R E C V A S G R O N I Q P P F E N
T A A E R O B I D N Y L K I G O N L O K C T K X T
G V A A N G A R I S T O S P A N T A P E S C O R N
I U O U S A L E T M O D T I I B T U D H T R P P L
A S O N B S O R P H Y D R O C O C O R T E F I O N
C W A C I N U C N K I X O P T O R I T A R N G I N
Y B P I X K U N L S I N E T A X A A Y B A I D L E
```

## Review questions

1.  Mrs. G. has been on glucocorticoid therapy for primary adrenal insufficiency. She has gained 7 lbs. and complains of being tired and depressed. Mrs. G. wants to stop taking the medication. Choose the best response:

    a.  "You must continue to take the medicine. If you stop taking the medicine, you will experience serious side effects."
    b.  "I know you are concerned about the weight gain and depression. I will speak with your physician to see how these problems can be improved."
    c.  "The doctor will decrease your dose and that should eliminate the side effects."
    d.  "You are right; it would be better to stop the medicine now before you have more serious side effects."

2.  Glucocorticosteroids cause an elevation in blood sugar because they

    a.  decrease the breakdown of adipose tissue.
    b.  suppress the inflammatory process.
    c.  decrease the utilization of glucose.
    d.  increase the rate at which new proteins are formed.

3.  When aldosterone is secreted, it causes

    a.  sodium to be excreted.
    b.  potassium to be excreted.
    c.  potassium to be reabsorbed.
    d.  hydrogen to be reabsorbed.

4.  When there is an excessive secretion of androgens in women, the following will result:

    a.  Amenorrhea.
    b.  Breast enlargement.
    c.  Anemia.
    d.  Excessive menses.

5.  A collagen disease treated with glucocorticosteroids is

    a.  Crohn's disease.
    b.  myasthenia gravis.
    c.  rheumatoid arthritis.
    d.  psoriasis.

6.  You are admitting Mr. J. who is to be started on corticosteroids. When you are taking Mr. J.'s history, he identifies that he has four diseases that have not previously been documented on the charts. For which one of the following would you contact the physician before starting the medication?

    a.  Atrial fibrillation.
    b.  Asthma.
    c.  Diabetes mellitus.
    d.  Epilepsy.

7.  The physician starts Mrs. R. on prednisone. You are to observe for Cushingoid syndrome, the symptoms of which are

    a.  hyperglycemia, polyuria, and poor wound healing.
    b.  "moon face," "buffalo hump," and thin extremities.
    c.  muscle weakness and muscle atrophy.
    d.  edema, hypertension, and hypokalemia.

8.  You know that your client who is taking dexamethasone (Decadron) understands the discharge teaching you have done if he states:

    a.  "I will contact the doctor if I get constipated or have diarrhea."
    b.  "I may lose my appetite so I will eat small, frequent meals."
    c.  "I will always take my medication on an empty stomach."
    d.  "I will weigh myself every week."

9.  Persons taking corticosteroids may want to increase their dietary intake of

    a.  sodium.
    b.  calcium.
    c.  chloride.
    d.  phosphorus.

10. Mr. H. is to use a beclomethasone (Vanceril) inhaler 1 t.i.d. Which of the following statements indicates that he needs additional teaching?

   a. "I will rinse my mouth after each use."
   b. "If I get a cold and sore throat, I will just use my inhaler four times a day."
   c. "I will shake the canister thoroughly before each use."
   d. "I will wait at least 1 minute between each breath."

## Critical thinking case study

K., age 9, is started on prednisone for glomerulonephritis because he has begun spilling protein in his urine.

1. Identify the instructions that you will give K.'s mother before he goes home.

K.'s mother asks you what she can expect as far as length of treatment, ongoing tests, etc.

2. Describe how you will respond to her questions.

You see K.'s mother 6 months later and she is in tears. She states that K. has gained 20 lbs. and that the children at school are making fun of her son and he is very unhappy.

3. Identify the best response to K.'s mother including any suggestions that would be helpful.

# CHAPTER 25

# Thyroid and Antithyroid Drugs

## Complete the following sentences

1. Production of $T_3$ and $T_4$ depends upon the presence of _____.

2. Thyroid hormone controls _____.

3. Thyroid hormones are required for _____ and _____.

4. The symptoms of adult hypothyroidism or _____ are _____ _____ and _____.

5. The CNS effects that a person with hyperthyroidism will exhibit are _____, _____, _____, _____, _____, and _____.

6. Thyroid storm or thyrotoxic crisis is characterized by _____, _____, _____, and _____.

7. Hyperthyroidism is treated by _____, _____, _____, or _____.

8. The drug of choice to treat hypothyroidism is _____ and it is administered _____ time(s) per day. The usual maintenance dose is _____ mg daily.

9. Propylthiouracil (Propacil) is used to treat _____.

10. An antiadrenergic drug used to treat cardiovascular conditions associated with hyperthyroidism is _____.

11. The normal values for $T_3$ are _____ and $T_4$ are_____.

12. Antithyroid drugs are administered for _____ months.

13. Children who are receiving thyroid replacement should have the following parameters monitored regularly: _____ and _____.

14. In older adults Synthroid should be held if the resting heart rate is greater than _____.

## Nursing Diagnosis

Identify three possible nursing diagnoses, pertinent assessment data, and nursing interventions associated with hyperthyroidism.

| Nursing Diagnoses | Assessment Data | Related Interventions |
|---|---|---|
| 1. | | |
| 2. | | |
| 3. | | |

**DEFINE:**

GOITER

CRETINISM

MYXEDEMA

THYROID STORM

## Review questions

1. After a thyroidectomy, your client is placed on Synthroid. Which of the following statements would indicate that your client needs further teaching?
   a. "I know that I will need periodic tests of thyroid function."
   b. "I will monitor my weight and pulse regularly."
   c. "When my symptoms subside, I will no longer need medication."
   d. "After my lab tests, my Synthroid dose may need to be changed."

2. Mr. J. has a blood work drawn. His $T_3$ is 0.05 and $T_4$ is 4 mg/100 ml. From the results of the lab work, you know that his medication dose
   a. needs to be increased.
   b. needs to be decreased.
   c. needs to be discontinued.
   d. is adequate.

3. People taking thyroid preparations should be observed for hyperthyroidism. Which of the following symptoms would be indicative of hyperthyroidism?
   a. Slow speech.
   b. Weight loss.
   c. Bradycardia.
   d. Decreased appetite.

4. Children who are receiving thyroid replacement should have which of the following parameters monitored regularly?

   a. Blood pressure.
   b. Fluid intake.

   c. Height and weight.
   d. Electrolytes.

5. Drugs that decrease the effects of thyroid hormones are

   a. antidepressants.
   b. anticonvulsants.

   c. anti-Parkinson's.
   d. antihypertensives.

6. An antiadrenergic drug used to treat cardiovascular symptoms in persons with hyperthyroidism is

   a. nifedipine (Procardia).
   b. propranolol (Inderal).

   c. verapamil (Calan).
   d. diltiazem (Cardizem).

7. The CNS symptom that a person with hyperthyroidism may exhibit is

   a. insomnia.
   b. lethargy.

   c. slow speech.
   d. hypoactive reflexes.

8. When administering a thyroid preparation, you should observe the client for changes in

   a. elimination.
   b. blood pressure.

   c. respiratory rate.
   d. heart rate.

9. A person with hyperthyroidism may have exophthalmos. Nursing measures that provide comfort include administering

   a. narcotic analgesics.
   b. lubricants.

   c. anti-inflammatory medications.
   d. sedatives.

10. Persons with hypothyroidism are especially sensitive to

    a. antihypertensives.
    b. steroids.

    c. diuretics.
    d. narcotics and sedatives.

## Critical thinking case study

Mrs. G, a 21-year-old female, has lost 10 lbs. since she was seen by her physician a year ago. She complains of headaches, insomnia, excessive perspiration, and constipation. Her vital signs are BP 100/60, pulse 120, resp. 16. Her physician diagnoses her with hyperthyroidism and starts her on propylthiouracil (Propacil) and propranolol (Inderal).

1. Identify which of Mrs. G's signs and symptoms are attributable to hyperthyroidism.

2. Explain to Mrs. G. why her physician ordered propranolol (Inderal) and propylthiouracil (Propacil), how long she will need to take the medications, and when she can expect to see the therapeutic effects from the medications.

3. Describe the instructions that you will give Mrs. G. regarding the adverse effects of the medications she is taking.

Two years after her initial treatment, Mrs. G. returns to the physician. She has gained 20 lbs. and complains of being tired. The physician orders thyroid function studies and finds them to be below the normal range. He starts Mrs. G. on .25 mg of Synthroid.

4. Identify why hypothyroidism must be treated.

5. Describe the instructions you will give Mrs. G. regarding Synthroid.

# CHAPTER 26

# Hormones That Regulate Calcium and Phosphorus Metabolism

## Complete the following sentences

1. Calcium and phosphorus metabolism is regulated by three hormones: _____, _____, and vitamin D.

2. Generally, when serum calcium levels go _____, serum phosphate levels go _____.

3. When calcium levels are low, the effect of the parathyroid hormone raises the level by acting on:
   a. bone to _____.
   b. intestine to _____.
   c. kidneys to _____.

4. Calcitonin _____ serum calcium levels by decreasing movement of calcium from _____ to _____. Its action is _____ but _____. It has little effect on _____calcium metabolism.

5. Vitamin D is obtained from _____ and _____. The main action of vitamin D is to raise _____ _____ by _____ intestinal absorption of dietary calcium and probably by _____.

6. Calcitriol (_____), a vitamin D preparation, is administered _____.

7. Deficiency of vitamin D causes inadequate absorption of _____ and _____.

8. The normal serum calcium level is _____.

9. Calcium is important in the regulation of
   a. _____.
   b. _____.
   c. _____.
   d. _____.
   e. _____.

10. Sources of calcium include _____, _____, and _____.

11. Factors that inhibit calcium absorption include _____, _____, _____ _____, _____ _____, _____.

12. Phosphorus is important because it

a. _____.

b. _____

c. _____.

d. _____.

e. _____.

13. Clinical manifestations of hypocalcemia are characterized by increased

_____ which may progress to _____.

14. Metabolic acidosis _____ the concentration of ionized calcium.

15. Two tests that help determine the presence of tetany are _____ sign and

_____ sign.

16. Calcium should be administered _____ meals.

17. A drug that increases the effect of calcium is _____.

18. Drugs that decrease the effect of calcium are _____, _____,

_____, _____, and _____.

19. _____ is a common cause of hypercalcemia.

20. Hypercalcemia can lead to calcium deposits in the kidneys which may lead to

_____ and _____.

21. Salmon calcitonin (Calcimar) _____ serum calcium levels.

22. Furosemide (_____) _____ calcium excretion in urine by preventing its reabsorption in renal tubules.

23. Hydrocortisone and prednisone antagonize effects of _____, therefore _____ intestinal absorption of calcium.

24. Plicamycin (Mithracin) lowers serum calcium by _____ _____.
A toxic effect of the drug is _____.

25. Normal saline inhibits

_____.

26. For clients experiencing hypercalcemia, fluids should be increased to _____ ml/day. Clients should drink cranberry juice to prevent the formation of _____.

## True or false

_____ 1. Everyone can benefit from calcium and vitamin D supplements.

_____ 2. Administration of laxatives can cause hypercalcemia.

_____ 3. If calcium is given to a digitalized client, the risks of digitalis toxicity increase.

_____ 4. Persons receiving anticonvulsant therapy are likely to develop hypercalcemia.

_____ 5. Oral calcium preparations should not be administered with tetracycline because they affect its absorption.

## Review questions

1. The demineralization of bone in rickets is caused by
   a. elevated calcium levels.
   b. a metastatic tumor.
   c. a vitamin D deficiency.
   d. the aging process.

2. Which of the following vitamins is administered with calcium to increase intestinal absorption of calcuim?
   a. vitamin A.
   b. vitamin $B_2$.
   c. vitamin C.
   d. vitamin D.

3. A person receiving phenytoin (Dilantin) therapy is likely to develop this side effect:
   a. hypercalcemia.
   b. hypocalcemia.
   c. hypophosphatemia.
   d. hyperkalemia.

4. Which of the following medications will cause increased serum calcium levels?
   a. Calcitonin-salmon (Calcimar).
   b. Calcitriol (Rocaltrol).
   c. Furosemide (Lasix).
   d. Plicamycin (Mithracin).

5. When a client is receiving calcium supplementation, for which of the following adverse effects should the nurse assess?
   a. Abdominal pain and constipation.
   b. Hypotension.
   c. Respiratory distress.
   d. Dizziness and syncope.

6. Ms. S. is diagnosed with osteoporosis. In addition to increasing her calcium, which of the following would be beneficial?
   a. Phosphorus supplements.
   b. Taking antacids with calcium supplements.
   c. Decreasing magnesium in her diet.
   d. Weight-bearing exercises.

7. When receiving feedback from Mrs. R. about her understanding of her calcium supplement regimen, which statement would lead you to believe that she understands the teaching that you have done?
   a. "I will take the medication with meals."
   b. "I will take the calcium with milk of magnesia to prevent constipation."
   c. "I will contact my physician if I feel weak or begin to urinate excessively."
   d. "I must limit my intake of foods high in vitamin D."

8. Mrs. H. is admitted with diabetic ketoacidosis. Which electrolyte imbalance is she likely to exhibit?
   a. Hypercalcemia.
   b. Hypocalcemia.
   c. Hyperphosphatemia.
   d. Hypokalemia.

9. Mrs. D. is admitted with an elevated serum calcium due to renal failure. She is started on prednisone 40 mg q.d., furosemide (Lasix) 40 mg b.i.d, and salmon calcitonin (Calcimar) 8 IU/kg q.i.d. If this treatment is effective, the next time her serum calcium is drawn, it should be
   a. 6.5–8 mg/100 ml.
   b. 8.5–10 mg/100 ml.
   c. 10.2–12.5 mg/100 ml.
   d. 12.7–14.5 mg/100 ml.

10. Mrs. S., a 75-year-old female, is being discharged after recovering from a fractured hip. Which instruction should be included when doing discharge teaching about prevention of hypocalcemia?
    a. Postmenopausal women who take estrogen need to take more calcium than women not taking estrogen.
    b. Everyone taking calcium also needs to take vitamin D supplements.
    c. You can use an inexpensive over-the-counter antacid called Tums which contains 200 mg calcium per tablet.
    d. You should use a calcium supplement that contains bone meal.

## Critical thinking case study

J.C., a 12-year-old male, is admitted to the hospital in acute renal failure.

Lab values:   creatinine  3.8
                     calcium    12.8 mg/100 ml
                     potassium  6.8

The physician orders: furosemide (Lasix) 40 mg IV, hydrocortisone (Solu Cortef) 40 mg IV, and 1000 cc 0.9% sodium chloride to run at 50 cc/hr. (The learner will need additional sources to answer the questions).

1.  Identify what you will be assessing for when J.C. is admitted.

2.  Discuss the rationale for the treatment plan.

A dual lumen catheter is inserted and J.C. is dialyzed. When J.C. returns from dialysis, he complains of a headache and nausea.

3.  Identify what you will do next.

J.C. is to continue to take furosemide (Lasix) once he returns home.

4.  Identify the teaching that you will do with J.C. and his mother to prepare him for discharge.

# CHAPTER 27

# Antidiabetic Agents

## Specify INCREASES or DECREASES

Insulin:

_____ 1. Storage of glycogen and fatty acids.

_____ 2. Breakdown of glucose.

_____ 3. Protein breakdown.

_____ 4. Protein and glycogen synthesis.

_____ 5. Production of glycerol and fatty acids.

_____ 6. Breakdown of fats.

_____ 7. Blood glucose levels.

## Matching exercise: terms and concepts

_____ 1. A type of hyperglycemia that occurs following an insulin-induced hypoglycemia reaction.

_____ 2. Changes in fatty subcutaneous tissue occurring from frequent injections.

_____ 3. Persons requiring large doses of insulin possibly due to the development of antibodies.

_____ 4. Symptoms include tachycardia, blurred vision, weakness, fatigue, and sweating.

_____ 5. This drug increases the effects of oral agents.

_____ 6. This drug raises blood glucose levels and antagonizes the effects of insulin.

_____ 7. The normal range for blood glucose levels.

_____ 8. Regular insulin peaks.

_____ 9. This test reflects the average blood sugar for 2–3 months.

_____ 10. A common complication that persons with diabetes experience.

A. Hyperglycemia.

B. MAO inhibitors.

C. Somogyi effect.

D. Lipodystrophy.

E. Allopurinol (Zyloprim).

F. Insulin resistance.

G. 80–130 mg/100 ml.

H. Hypoglycemia.

I. Oral contraceptives.

J. 60–100 mg/100 ml.

K. 2–3 hours.

L. 4–6 hours.

M. Glycosylated hemoglobin.

N. Urinary tract infections.

## True or false

_____ 1. Early symptoms of diabetic ketoacidosis include blurred vision, anorexia, nausea, vomiting, thirst, and polyuria.

_____ 2. Insulin can be stored at room temperature.

_____ 3. Type II diabetics require only oral agents to control their diabetes mellitus.

_____ 4. Oral agents are contraindicated during pregnancy.

_____ 5. Once insulin has been started, the person will remain on the medication the rest of his or her life.

_____ 6. Symptoms of hypoglycemia include excessive thirst, hunger, and increased urine output.

_____ 7. Salicylates taken with antidiabetic drugs increase the likelihood of hypoglycemia.

_____ 8. Persons taking adrenocorticosteroids and thiazide diuretics will require less insulin.

_____ 9. Insulin is necessary for normal growth and development in children.

_____ 10. When treating hypoglycemia, the primary goal is to restore the brain's supply of glucose.

_____ 11. A honeymoon period, characterized by recovery of islet function and temporary production of insulin, may occur after diabetes is first diagnosed and treated.

_____ 12. Once hypoglycemia is relieved, the client should consume foods high in fat to replace glycogen stores and prevent secondary hypoglycemia.

## Crossword puzzle

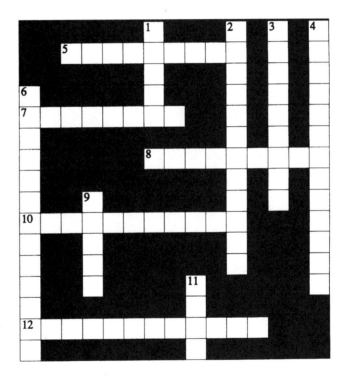

**Across**

5. A second-generation sulfonylurea, recommended for patients with impaired renal function.
7. One of the preferred types of insulin for long-term therapy.
8. This oral antidiabetic drug has a diuretic effect.
10. These drugs with insulin can increase the chance of hypoglycemia.
12. This reaction to insulin includes tachycardia, hunger, muscle tremors, and blurred vision.

**Down**

1. This type of insulin is preferred for poorly controlled diabetes.
2. Isotonic IV fluids are an important part of treating diabetic _____.
3. A useful drug for diabetics who have fluid retention and edema.
4. Preferred oral hypoglycemic for diabetics with gout.
6. Failing to change insulin injection sites can lead to this.
9. Lack of insulin leads to high blood _____ levels.
11. Insulin from this source is the most antigenic type.

## Review questions

1. Mr. J.'s blood glucose report is 40 mg/100 ml. This value is
   a. below the normal range.
   b. within the normal range.
   c. above the normal range.

2. Mr. J. asks you why he must receive insulin by injection. The best explanation would be that
   a. adequate insulin levels cannot be achieved orally.
   b. enzymes in the gastrointestinal tract destroy insulin.
   c. injections promote endogenous production of insulin.
   d. oral preparations deteriorate quickly and cannot be stored.

3. J. receives 30 units of NPH insulin at 8 A.M. At what time of day should the nurse be alert for a potential hypoglycemic reaction?
   a. After breakfast.
   b. After lunch.
   c. Before bedtime.
   d. Before dinner.

4. Which of the following statements by M. leads you to believe that she has a good understanding of insulin administration?
   a. "Regular insulin is drawn up first, then NPH insulin."
   b. "Two units of air should be drawn up in each syringe."
   c. "Insulin that has a precipitant should not be used."
   d. "The insulin should be shaken well before I draw it up."

5. K. is 10 years old and a newly diagnosed type I diabetic. K is at high risk for
   a. decreased cardiac output.
   b. fluid volume excess.
   c. altered nutrition less than body requirement.
   d. alteration in growth and development.

6. When teaching J. about the early signs and symptoms of hypoglycemia, you tell him he may experience
   a. sweating.
   b. polyuria.
   c. polydipsia.
   d. dizziness.

7. Mr. H. is started on glyburide (Diabeta). Patient teaching should include the following information:
   a. Exercise should be avoided until you have been on the medication 2 months.
   b. Always take the medication with milk.
   c. You do not have to adhere to regular meal times.
   d. Headaches and lethargy are indicative of hypoglycemia.

8. The physician may order which of the following lab studies to evaluate compliance with medication, diet, and exercise regimen?
   a. Serum glucose.
   b. Routine urine.
   c. Glycosylated hemoglobin.
   d. Serum creatinine.

9. When doing teaching with diabetic clients, it is important that they understand that poor blood sugar control leads to the development of atherosclerosis because of
   a. increased conversion of fatty acids to cholesterol.
   b. decreased rate of gluconeogenesis.
   c. increased production of fatty acids.
   d. decreased breakdown of glucose.

10. You know that Mrs. J. has understood the teaching that you have done regarding glipizide (Glucotrol) if she states that glipizide (Glucotrol)
    a. increases the peripheral uptake of glucose.
    b. decreases the body's need for insulin.
    c. increases hepatic glucose production.
    d. stimulates beta cells in the pancreas.

## Critical thinking case study

Mrs. J. is a 25-year-old married woman newly diagnosed with type I diabetes mellitus. She takes 3 units Reg. Humulin Insulin and 14 units NPH Humulin Insulin in A.M. and 4 units Reg and 10 units NPH before dinner.

One month after starting the regime, she comes to the emergency room with confusion, tremor, and tachycardia. The physician diagnoses her with hypoglycemia and starts intravenous glucose. When you interview Mrs. J., you discover that she had influenza and had been unable to eat.

1. Identify the information that you will share with Mrs. J. and her husband about diet and lifestyle changes that would help her control her diabetes.

2. Identify what information you will review with Mrs. J. that will help her manage her insulin therapy.

One month after discharge, Mr. J. calls you and states that his wife is unresponsive and asks you what to do.

3. Discuss your response to Mr. J.

# CHAPTER 28

# Estrogens, Progestins, and Oral Contraceptives

## True or false

_____ 1. The use of estrogen may aggravate gallbladder disease.

_____ 2. Persons taking estrogen will need phosphorus supplementation.

_____ 3. Progesterone stimulates milk production.

_____ 4. Estrogen has been used to prevent excessive height in young girls.

_____ 5. During pregnancy the placenta produces large amounts of estrogen.

_____ 6. One of the problems associated with estrogen is fluid volume deficit and hyponatremia.

_____ 7. Progesterone decreases uterine motility.

_____ 8. Women with diabetes mellitus may not use birth control pills.

_____ 9. Diethylstilbestrol (Stilbestrol) is the only estrogen approved as a postcoital contraceptive.

_____ 10. Estrogen and progestins should be taken on an empty stomach.

_____ 11. Birth control pills are used in the treatment of amenorrhea.

_____ 12. Estrogen is administered after delivery to suppress lactation.

_____ 13. Acne is a common adverse effect of taking birth control pills.

_____ 14. Birth control pills may only be taken for 5 years.

_____ 15. Progestins reduce the risk of endometrial cancer in women.

## Name that drug

_____ 1. Administered via patch, worn three consecutive weeks a month.

_____ 2. Used topically for atrophic or senile vaginitis.

_____ 3. Administered twice a day for five days for postcoital contraception.

_____ 4. Can be administered intravenously for dysfunctional uterine bleeding.

_____ 5. Administered IM at the end of the first stage of labor to prevent postpartum breast engorgement.

_____ 6. Given IM in 1.5–2 mg doses once a month to treat female hypogonadism.

_____ 7. Given IM once every 4 weeks times 4 doses for amenorrhea or dysfunctional bleeding.

_____ 8. Used for endometrial cancer, administered IM weekly until improvement, then monthly.

_____ 9. A commonly prescribed estrogen used for treatment of menopause.

_____ 10. A drug used to prevent osteoporosis in postmenopausal women.

_____ 11. These drugs decrease the effects of oral anticoagulants, insulin, oral antidiabetic agents, and antihypertensive drugs.

_____ 12. Used to treat ovarian failure.

_____ 13. Used to test estrogen production.

_____ 14. An oral contraceptive that contains no estrogen.

_____ 15. If this aminoglycoside is administered with oral contraceptives, it will decrease their effectiveness.

## Review questions

1. Persons using birth control pills are at risk for developing blood clots because estrogen
   a. increases serum triglycerides, cholesterol, and glucose.
   b. stimulates skeletal growth, causing increased production of red blood cells.
   c. increases blood levels of several clotting factors.
   d. causes peripheral vasoconstriction.

2. Mr. B., a 76-year-old male, is started on estrogen for metastatic prostatic cancer. Which of the following statements by Mr. B. leads you to believe that he needs further teaching?
   a. "The doctor will check my blood sugar on a routine basis."
   b. "I may experience impotence which will subside when the drug is stopped."
   c. "I will not become alarmed if my breasts enlarge."
   d. "I will take this medication for the rest of my life."

3. Mrs. K. is a 33-year-old mother of two with a history of asthma and migraine headaches. She is on a low-residue diet for colitis. Which of the factors in Mrs. K.'s history would contraindicate the use of birth control pills?
   a. Migraine headaches.
   b. Age.
   c. Asthma.
   d. Colitis.

4. Estradiol (Estraderm) is administered to postmenopausal women to prevent
   a. endometriosis.
   b. dysfunctional uterine bleeding.
   c. osteoporosis.
   d. uterine cancer.

5. Which of the following medications is administered to stop dysfunctional uterine bleeding?
   a. Estropipate (Ogen).
   b. Medroxyprogesterone acetate (Depo-Provera).
   c. Ethinyl estradiol (Estinyl).
   d. Polyestradiol phosphate (Estradurin).

6. Ms. H. is to be started on birth control pills. Which of the following statements indicates that she needs additional teaching?
   a. "I will monitor my weight and have my blood pressure checked monthly."
   b. "I will have a pap smear done on a yearly basis."
   c. "I will continue to do monthly self-breast examination even though these pills should decrease my risk for developing breast cancer."
   d. "I know nausea is common so I will make sure that I take the medication at the same time each day with food."

7. Which of the following statements by Mrs. G. leads you to believe that she has a good understanding of how to take Nelova 10/11?
   a. "I will take the medication for 3 weeks and a placebo for a week."
   b. "I will take a pill every morning and evening."
   c. "If I miss a pill I will not take 2 the next day."
   d. "If I experience break-through bleeding, I should immediately stop the medication."

8. Which of the following medications, when administered concurrently with oral contraceptives, will decrease their effect?

   a. Anticonvulsants.

   b. Antihypertensives.

   c. Anticoagulants.

   d. Anticholinergics.

9. Which of the following instructions should be included when you are teaching someone about transdermal estrogen?

   a. Apply the patches to the chest and upper back only.

   b. The patches are irritating so apply a thin layer of medicated cream before application of the patch.

   c. The patch should be applied in the morning and taken off at bedtime.

   d. Change the patches every 3 to 4 days.

10. Persons taking estrogen need to be assessed regularly for the following adverse effect:

    a. Hypoglycemia.

    b. Weight loss.

    c. Hypertension.

    d. Arrhythmias.

## Critical thinking case study

Mrs. G. has come to the gynecologist requesting birth control pills.

1. Identify what factors would contraindicate the use of birth control pills and why.

2. Identify the assessments that should be done before birth control is started.

Ms. G. calls you after taking birth control pills for 2 months, stating that she has severe acne and has gained 5 pounds.

3. Identify your response to Mrs. G.

Ms. G. returns to the office 1 year after starting on birth control pills. Ms. G. complains of leg pain.

4.  Identify what you will do.

# CHAPTER 29

# Androgens and Anabolic Steroids

## Circle the correct answer

1. There will be a/an increase/decrease of skin thickness when androgens/anabolic steroids are administered.

2. With the administration of androgens/anabolic steroids, protein anabolism increases/decreases and protein catabolism increases/decreases.

3. When anabolic steroids are administered, there is a(an) increased/decreased secretion of FSH, LH, and ICSH.

4. When anabolic steroids are administered to women, they increase/decrease the lining of the uterus.

5. Persons taking androgens/anabolic steroids will notice a(an) increase/decrease in muscle mass.

6. When androgens are administered to young children, the result will be a significant increase/decrease in growth.

7. Androgens increase/decrease the development of female sexual characteristics.

8. When androgens/anabolic steroids are administered, there will be a(an) increased/decreased body weight.

9. When anabolic steroids are administered to adult males, the result will be a(an) increased/ decreased sperm count.

10. Androgens/anabolic steroids will increase/decrease appetite.

11. Administration of androgens/anabolic steroids results in a(an) increase/decrease in sodium and water retention.

12. Administration of anabolic steroids increases/decreases the risk of developing prostatic cancer.

13. When a person takes antihistamines with anabolic steroids, there will be a(an) increase/decrease in the effect of the steroids.

14. Persons taking anabolic steroids have documented a(an) increase/decrease in body hair.

15. Androgens/anabolic steroids increase/decrease hematocrit and hemoglobin levels.

## Crossword puzzle

### Across

2. This drug's dosage may need to be decreased during androgen treatment.
3. One dangerous side effect of anabolic steroid use is an _____ imbalance.
5. Androgen therapy in children can lead to premature _____ closure.
6. For short-term treatment of postpartum breast engorgement.
7. Administered to younger males with cryptorchidism.
8. A hormone that stimulates testosterone secretion.
9. Used in the treatment of osteoporosis.

### Down

1. Used to treat endometriosis and fibrocystic breast disease.
3. This type of androgen may be given orally.
4. Produced in the human body by Leydig's cells.

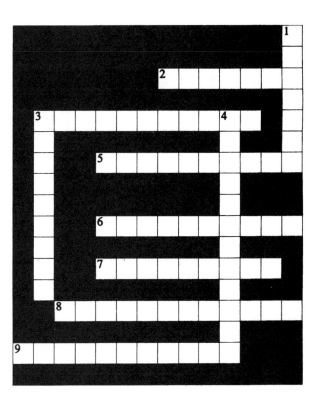

## Review questions

1. Which of the following medications, if administered concurrently with anabolic steroids, will decrease their effects?
   - a. Beta adrenergic blockers.
   - b. Antihistamines.
   - c. Thiazide diuretics.
   - d. Cholinergic drugs.

2. Persons taking anabolic steroids may experience which of the following adverse effects?
   - a. Elevated blood urea nitrogen.
   - b. Elevated blood sugar.
   - c. Bradycardia.
   - d. Hypertension.

3. Physical changes that occur with the use of anabolic steroids in males include
   - a. thinning of skin.
   - b. increased sperm count.
   - c. rapid bone growth.
   - d. increased endurance.

4. When androgens are administered to adult females, the following can result:
   - a. Atrophy of breasts.
   - b. Rapid bone growth.
   - c. Loss of pubic hair.
   - d. Suppression of menstruation.

5. Nandrolone decanoate (Deca-Durabolin) is administered to adult females to prevent
   - a. endometriosis.
   - b. fibrocystic breast disease.
   - c. postpartum breast engorgement.
   - d. osteoporosis.

6. Mr. J.'s physician starts him on androgens for treatment of impotence. Which of the following statements by Mr. J. leads you to believe that he has understood the teaching that you have done?

   a. "If I experience increasing baldness, I will contact my physician immediately."

   b. "If my skin appears yellow or my urine turns dark, I will contact my physician."

   c. "I know that my red blood count may drop so I will look for bruising and contact my physician if I see any."

   d. "I know that headaches are common with this drug so I will not become alarmed if I have a severe headache."

7. Mrs. A. is receiving methyltestosterone (Metandren) for advanced breast cancer. Which of the following electrolyte disturbances should you be assessing for?

   a. Hyponatremia.

   b. Hypokalemia.

   c. Hypercalcemia.

   d. Hyperchloremia.

8. When nandrolone phenpropionate (Durabolin) is ordered for the treatment of anemia, it should be given with

   a. folic acid.

   b. iron.

   c. thiamine.

   d. vitamin $B_{12}$.

9. Mrs. H. is receiving nandrolone phenpropionate (Durabolin) for breast cancer. An expected outcome resulting from the administration of this medication is

   a. decreased calcium levels.

   b. decreased pain.

   c. decreased edema.

   d. decreased nausea and vomiting.

10. Androgens potentiate the effect of the following medications. Therefore, the dose of which drugs may need to be decreased while persons are receiving androgen therapy?

   a. Calcium channel blockers.

   b. Oral antidiabetic agents.

   c. Loop diuretics.

   d. Anticholinergic drugs.

## Critical thinking case study

You are the school nurse at East Side High School. The wrestling coach asks you to give a presentation on anabolic steroids.

1. Develop a presentation that would convince teenage boys not to use anabolic steroids.

2. Identify ways the school nurse can monitor the health of high school athletes and possibly detect the use of steroids.

# SECTION V

# Nutrients, Fluids, and Electrolytes

---

## CHAPTER 30

## Nutritional Products, Anorexiants, and Digestants

### Fill in the blank

Place a *P* for protein, a *C* for carbohydrate, a *W* for water, or an *F* for fat next to each body function.

_____ 1. Furnishes amino acids.

_____ 2. Helps maintain body temperature.

_____ 3. Promotes normal function of nerve cells.

_____ 4. Assists in maintaining normal osmotic pressure.

_____ 5. Transports nutrients to body cells.

_____ 6. Promotes normal fat metabolism.

_____ 7. Helps maintain electrolyte balance.

_____ 8. Promotes bowel elimination.

_____ 9. Protects organs from injury.

_____ 10. Promotes normal growth and development.

### True or false

_____ 1. An increased hematocrit is indicative of fluid volume excess.

_____ 2. Persons with a water excess will have a low serum sodium and may experience disorientation.

_____ 3. Persons with a protein deficit will be in metabolic alkalosis.

_____ 4. Persons with a poor protein intake may have edema.

_____ 5. Persons who are obese are more susceptible to developing an infection.

_____ 6. Tube feedings are better tolerated if they are diluted initially.

_____ 7. Intermittent feedings are preferable because diarrhea and gastric distention are decreased.

_____ 8. A nasogastric tube will prevent the complication of aspiration.

_____ 9. Pancreatic enzymes should be administered with food.

_____ 10. Cold tube feedings are better tolerated than those at room temperature.

## Matching exercise: terms and concepts

Match the formula or elemental diet with the population for which it is intended.

_____ 1. Portagen.

_____ 2. Pulmocare.

_____ 3. Nutramigen.

_____ 4. Flexical.

_____ 5. Isomil.

_____ 6. Pregestimil.

_____ 7. Vivonex.

A. Infants with malabsorption syndromes.

B. Persons with chronic obstructive pulmonary disease.

C. Persons with fat and malabsorption problems.

D. Persons with GI disorders because it requires no digestion and leaves no fecal residue.

E. Persons allergic to milk.

F. Children who are allergic to ordinary proteins.

G. Persons who have had bowel surgery.

## Complete the following sentences

1. The most commonly used dextrose solution is _____ which provides _____ Kcal/liter.

2. For total parenteral nutrition _____ and _____ solutions are used. They are _____ and so they must be given through a central line.

3. Five hundred milliliters of a 10% fat emulsion provides _____ calories.

4. When a person is receiving tube feedings, additional _____ is necessary between feedings.

5. Most tube feedings are _____ and will therefore _____ fluid volume deficit if water is not administered with them.

6. TPN or hyperalimentation contains _____ and _____.

7. Fat emulsions provide _____ and can be administered _____.

8. Before administering a tube feeding, the nurse should check _____.

9. The maximum amount of tube feeding, including water, that should be administered at any one time is _____.

10. Clients receiving 2000 cc/day of tube feeding should receive _____ ml of water.

## Review questions

1. A 1000 ml of D5W provides
   a. 170 calories.
   b. 200 calories.
   c. 300 calories.
   d. 500 calories.

2. An electrolyte imbalance that can result from administering hypertonic solutions is
   a. hypokalemia.
   b. hyperkalemia.
   c. hyponatremia.
   d. hypernatremia.

3. An expected outcome for Mr. C., who is being treated with IV fluids for severe dehydration, would be
   a. a drop in blood pressure.
   b. a drop in hematocrit.
   c. an increase in serum sodium.
   d. an increased serum potassium level.

4. Which of the following statements by your client would lead you to believe that she has understood the teaching that you have done about pancreatin, a pancreatic enzyme?

   a. "I will take the pancreatin on an empty stomach."

   b. "I will increase the fat in my diet."

   c. "I will take the pancreatin with meals."

   d. "I will increase foods high in vitamin C in my diet."

5. Which of the following liquid formulas is the most appropriate for a baby who is allergic to ordinary food proteins?

   a. Portagen.

   b. PediaSure.

   c. Pregestimil.

   d. Nutramigen.

6. Persons receiving anorexiant drugs to decrease appetite should be instructed that they are only effective for

   a. 1–2 weeks.

   b. 4–6 weeks.

   c. 2–3 months.

   d. 4–6 months.

7. Phenylpropanolamine, an ingredient in Dexatrim, may produce the following disorder:

   a. Edema.

   b. Migraine headaches.

   c. Hypertension.

   d. Diabetes mellitus.

8. Total parenteral nutrition (TPN)

   a. may cause a fluid deficit and metabolic acidosis.

   b. provides essential fatty acids.

   c. provides carbohydrates and amino acids.

   d. may lower serum sodium levels.

9. Mr. J. is admitted from home with confusion. The following are the results of his blood studies: Na+ 118, K+ 3.5, glucose 80. After analyzing his blood study results, which electrolyte imbalance would you suspect is contributing to his confusion?

   a. Hyponatremia.

   b. Hypernatremia.

   c. Hypokalemia.

   d. Hypoglycemia.

10. Mr. J., who has a 15-year history of chronic obstructive pulmonary disease, is to receive Pulmocare for his supplemental feedings because

    a. it promotes healing.

    b. its metabolism produces less carbon dioxide.

    c. it is high in nitrogen and high in carbohydrates.

    d. it requires no digestion and leaves no fecal residue.

## Crtitical thinking case study

Mr. J. is a 76-year-old man with a 10-year history of COPD. His most recent hospital admission is for a cerebral vascular accident. He is unresponsive and has a large pressure sore on his coccyx. A nasogastric tube is inserted and he is to receive 80 ml of Pulmocare every hour in continuous feedings.

1. Identify why Pulmocare was chosen for the supplemental feeding for Mr. J.

2. Identify the nursing assessment that you will do for Mr. J.

3. Discuss the advantages and disadvantages of TPN and enteral feedings and identify why Mr. J. was started on tube feeding instead of TPN.

4. Identify potential problems that a client with a tube feeding can experience and how these problems can be avoided.

Mr. J. experiences diarrhea four times during your shift.

5. Identify your nursing actions.

# CHAPTER 31

# Vitamins

## Matching exercise: terms and concepts

_____ 1. Required for normal vision.

_____ 2. Found in cereals, green vegetables, egg yolks, and vegetable oils.

_____ 3. Essential for normal clotting.

_____ 4. Essential in fat and carbohydrate metabolism.

_____ 5. Necessary for the normal development of RBCs and for growth.

_____ 6. Found in liver, kidney beans, and green vegetables.

_____ 7. Essential for fat synthesis.

_____ 8. Necessary for synthesis of cholesterol.

_____ 9. Helps maintain cellular immunity.

_____ 10. May function in the production of corticosteroids.

_____ 11. Found in dried beans, whole grains, and peanuts.

_____ 12. Not stored in body to a significant extent; excess is excreted in the urine.

_____ 13. Fat-soluble vitamin obtained from exposure of skin to sunlight.

A. Folic acid (folate).

B. Niacin (vitamin $B_3$).

C. Riboflavin (vitamin $B_2$).

D. Vitamin A.

E. Pantothenic acid (vitamin $B_5$).

F. Vitamin E.

G. Thiamine (vitamin $B_1$).

H. Vitamin K.

I. Pyridoxine (vitamin $B_6$).

J. Biotin.

K. Vitamin D.

L. Cyanocobalamin (vitamin $B_{12}$).

M. Vitamin C (ascorbic acid).

## Name the deficiency/excess

_____ 1. Causes night blindness.

_____ 2. Results in bleeding abnormalities.

_____ 3. Symptoms include anorexia, nausea, depression, and muscle pain.

_____ 4. Causes convulsions, peripheral neuritis, and mental depression.

_____ 5. Can cause renal calculi.

_____ 6. Causes Wernicke–Korsakoff syndrome.

_____ 7. Neurologic symptoms of this disorder include paresthesia, unsteady gait, and depressed deep tendon reflexes.

_____ 8. Can cause scurvy.

_____ 9. Causes impaired growth in children.

_____ 10. Increases intracranial pressure.

_____ 11. May be caused by smoking.

_____ 12. Causes eye disorders (burning, itching, photophobia).

_____ 13. Causes delusions, hallucinations, and impaired peripheral motor function.

_____ 14. Can increase the amounts of oxalate in urine.

_____ 15. Causes pernicious anemia.

_____ 16. Results from a lack of hydrochloric acid or intrinsic factor in the stomach.

_____ 17. Occurs commonly in newborns.

_____ 18. Early manifestations include anorexia, vomiting, irritability, and skin changes.

_____ 19. Alcoholism is a common cause.

_____ 20. Persons using oral contraceptives are at risk for developing this.

## Review questions

1. Persons who smoke cigarettes are at risk for developing a deficiency of which of the following vitamins?

   a. Vitamin A.
   b. Vitamin $B_6$.

   c. Vitamin C.
   d. Vitamin D.

2. Mrs. J. has multiple sclerosis and has an indwelling catheter. Which of the following vitamins should you recommend that she take to acidify her urine and thereby help decrease her likelihood of developing a urinary tract infection?

   a. Folic acid (folate).
   b. Pantothenic acid (vitamin $B_5$).

   c. Niacin (nicotinic acid).
   d. Vitamin C (ascorbic acid).

3. Persons taking oral contraceptives need to be instructed to increase the following vitamin in their diet:

   a. Vitamin K.
   b. Vitamin C.

   c. Vitamin D.
   d. Riboflavin (vitamin $B_2$).

4. Mrs. B. is started on vitamin $B_{12}$ for pernicious anemia. An expected outcome of the administration of this medication is

   a. decreased bleeding.
   b. increased hematocrit.

   c. decreased joint pain.
   d. improved vision.

5. Mr. X. is started on oral niacin to decrease his cholesterol. Which of the following adverse reactions should you be observing for?

   a. Hypotension.
   b. Tachycardia.

   c. Nose bleeds.
   d. Diarrhea.

6. Mr. H., a 59-year-old truck driver, is experiencing night blindness. An increase in which one of the following vitamins may help improve his vision?

   a. Vitamin A.
   b. Vitamin $B_2$.

   c. Vitamin C.
   d. Vitamin D.

7. Mrs. J. is started on Coumadin and instructed to avoid foods high in vitamin K. These include

   a. carrots, potatoes, squash.
   b. apricots, peaches, cantaloupe.

   c. meat, whole milk, margarine.
   d. green leafy vegetables, wheat bran.

8. Mrs. H. is experiencing anorexia, vomiting, headache, and fatigue. An excess of which of the following vitamins can cause these symptoms?

   a. Vitamin A.
   b. Vitamin $B_{12}$.

   c. Vitamin C.
   d. Vitamin D.

9. Mrs. C., who has pernicious anemia, asks you why vitamin $B_{12}$ must be administered parenterally. The best response to her question is that

   a. the intrinsic factor in your stomach that is required for absorption of vitamin $B_{12}$ is absent.

   b. oral ingestion of vitamin $B_{12}$ causes irritation and bleeding.

   c. pernicious anemia causes changes in the mucous membrane lining and impairs absorption.

   d. with severe deficiencies like yours, oral vitamin $B_{12}$ is not effective.

10. Mr. C. complains of headaches, dizziness, insomnia, and depression. He may require supplementation of which of the following vitamins to correct these symptoms?

   a. Pyridoxine (vitamin $B_6$).

   b. Pantothenic acid (vitamin $B_5$).

   c. Niacin (vitamin $B_3$).

   d. Riboflavin (vitamin $B_2$).

## Critical thinking case study

Mr. J., a severely malnourished 76-year-old alcoholic, is admitted to your unit. Mr. J.'s physician orders niacin (vitamin $B_3$), thiamine (vitamin $B_1$), and folic acid (folate) to be administered by IM injection.

1. Specify the nursing assessments that you will do (including analysis of lab studies) when Mr. J. is admitted.

2. Discuss the rationale for using these medications and why they are administered parenterally.

Two days after admission, Mr. J. states, "I will not take any more shots and that is final."

3. Discuss how you will proceed.

# CHAPTER 32

# Minerals and Electrolytes

## Matching exercise: terms and concepts

_____ 1. Necessary for normal cell growth and synthesis of carbohydrates and proteins.

_____ 2. Essential component of hemoglobin.

_____ 3. Causes skeletal muscle weakness, respiratory insufficiency, and drowsiness.

_____ 4. Causes abdominal distension, constipation, and paralytic ileus.

_____ 5. This trace element is found in seafood.

_____ 6. Strengthens bones by promoting calcium retention.

_____ 7. This trace element is found in brain, heart, liver, kidneys, bone, and muscle.

_____ 8. A component of vitamin $B_{12}$ that is required for normal function of all body cells.

_____ 9. Symptoms include headache, dizziness, weakness, lethargy, restlessness, confusion, convulsions.

_____ 10. An exchange resin used for the treatment of hypokalemia.

_____ 11. A chelating agent used to remove excess iron.

_____ 12. Increases the effectiveness of insulin.

_____ 13. Assists in regulating osmotic pressure.

_____ 14. Eliminated from the body primarily by the kidneys.

_____ 15. Shifts in and out of the red blood cells in exchange for bicarbonate.

A. Copper.

B. Hyponatremia.

C. Deferoxamine (Desferal Mesylate).

D. Hypermagnesemia.

E. Chromium.

F. Iron.

G. Zinc.

H. Hypokalemia.

I. Fluoride.

J. Sodium.

K. Cobalt.

L. Potassium.

M. Iodine.

N. Magnesium.

O. Chloride.

P. Sodium polystyrene sulfonate (Kayexalate).

## Name that imbalance

_____ 1. Causes peaked T waves, prolonged P-R intervals, and prolonged QRS complexes.

_____ 2. Signs and symptoms include impaired growth, anorexia, loss of taste and smell, and poor wound healing.

_____ 3. Results in increased extracellular volume.

_____ 4. Occurs in women who take oral contraceptives.

_____ 5. Can occur as a result of acidosis.

_____ 6. Produces impaired glucose tolerance and impaired growth and reproduction.

_____ 7. Causes depressed ST segments and inverted T waves.

_____ 8. Menkes syndrome is caused by this.

_____ 9. Hypotension is a symptom of this.

_____ 10. Results in bronze pigmentation of the skin.

_____ 11. Hyperaldosteronism and Cushing's disease can cause this.

_____ 12. Results in impaired erythropoiesis.

_____ 13. Can result from overhydration and swelling of brain cells.

_____ 14. Results in skeletal muscle weakness and paralysis.

_____ 15. Impairs carbohydrate metabolism and decreases secretion of insulin.

_____ 16. Excessive administration of ammonium chloride can cause this.

_____ 17. Muscle spasms and tetany can result from this.

_____ 18. Administration of large amounts of penicillin G can cause this.

_____ 19. Commonly occurs with alcoholism.

_____ 20. Causes depressant effects on the neuromuscular system.

## Review questions

1. Copper is a trace element important
   a. for cell growth and synthesis of carbohydrates.
   b. because it increases the effectiveness of insulin.
   c. because it assists in regulating osmotic pressure.
   d. in the formation of red blood cells.

2. Mr. J. is admitted with dehydration. His lab values are: $Na^+$ 155 mEq/liter, $K^+$ 5 mEq/l, $Cl^-$ 100mEq/l, $Mg^{++}$ 2.0 mEq/l. Identify the electrolyte imbalance that Mr. J. is experiencing.
   a. Hypernatremia.
   b. Hyperkalemia.
   c. Hypochloremia.
   d. Hypomagnesemia.

3. Sodium polystyrene sulfonate (Kayexalate) is administered for the treatment of
   a. hypokalemia.
   b. hyperkalemia.
   c. hyponatremia.
   d. hypernatremia.

4. Excessive ingestion of iron can result in
   a. heart failure.
   b. respiratory failure.
   c. encephalopathy.
   d. renal failure.

5. Zinc can be found in
   a. citrus fruits.
   b. milk and yogurt.
   c. wheat germ.
   d. green leafy vegetables.

6. An iodine deficiency can cause
   a. thyroid enlargement.
   b. myocardial enlargement.
   c. stomatitis.
   d. lymphadenopathy.

7. Mrs. G. is being discharged on an iron supplement. Which of the following statements by Mrs. G. indicates that she understands the teaching that you have done?
   a. "If my stool becomes dark, I will contact my physician immediately."
   b. "I can take the iron with vitamin C to increase its absorption."
   c. "I can only take the medication an hour before meals."
   d. "I can expect an increase in my appetite in about a week."

8. Symptoms of hyponatremia that the nurse needs to observe for when loop diuretics are administered, include
   a. bradycardia.
   b. diarrhea.
   c. respiratory insufficiency.
   d. confusion.

9. Instructions that a client who is being discharged on potassium supplements should receive:

   a. Take the medication on a full stomach.
   b. If you need diuretics for any reason, you should use a potassium sparing diuretic.
   c. The medication should be taken with milk, not juice.
   d. Do not use salt, but you may use salt substitute.

10. Excessive use of cathartics can produce a magnesium excess. A client with hypermagnesemia should be observed for

    a. paralytic ileus.
    b. hypertension.
    c. respiratory insufficiency.
    d. seizures.

## Critical thinking case study

Mr. B. is seen in the emergency room for chest pain. He has not been feeling well for some time. He has been treated for hypertension for 5 years. His blood pressure is 170/90 and pulse is 110.

Laboratory values are:  BUN 108 mg/dl
                       creatinine 10 mg/dl
                       sodium 142 mEq/l
                       potassium 7 mEq/l

1. Identify and prioritize your nursing actions.

The physician diagnoses Mr. B. with renal failure and orders sodium bicarbonate 45 mEq over 15 minutes and 5 ml of 10% calcium gluconate.

2. Identify what you will be assessing for.

Mr. B.'s potassium comes down to 5.9 mEq/l. His physician orders Kayexelate in sorbitol via enema. Mr. B. asks you why the medication must be administered this way.

3. Describe how you will respond to Mr. B's inquiry.

# SECTION VI

# Drugs Used to Treat Infections

---

## CHAPTER 33

## General Characteristics of Anti-infective Drugs

---

## Complete the following sentences

1. Factors that predispose one to infection include

   a. _____.

   b. _____.

   c. _____.

   d. _____.

   e. _____.

   f. _____.

   g. _____.

   h. _____.

   i. _____.

2. A hospital-acquired infection is also referred to as a _____ infection.

3. Antimicrobial drugs include _____, _____, and _____.

4. The term _____ refers to killing of micro-organisms.

5. The term _____ refers to inhibition of growth of microorganisms.

6. For most acute infections, the average duration of treatment with an antibiotic is _____ days.

7. If your client has renal insufficiency, the dose of the antibiotic may need to be _____.
   The drug dosage is based on the individual's _____ clearance.

8. Drugs that may cause nephrotoxicity and ototoxicity include _____.

9. Most oral anti-infectives should be given _____ before meals with _____ ounces of $H_2O$.

10. Adverse effects of antibiotics that the nurse should observe for include _____,
    _____, _____, and _____.

11. Common symptoms that can be seen with a super infection are:

    a. _____.

    b. _____.

    c. _____.

    d. _____.

    e. _____.

## Review questions

1. All of the following factors predispose a person to infection *except*
   a. impaired blood supply.
   b. hypertension.
   c. suppression of immune system.
   d. advanced age.

2. Anti-infective drugs work in the following ways:
   a. Enhancing cell metabolism and growth.
   b. Promoting protein synthesis.
   c. Inhibiting cell wall synthesis.
   d. Stimulating bacterial reproduction.

3. If your client has renal insufficiency, the dose of antibiotic ordered should be
   a. increased.
   b. decreased.
   c. unchanged.
   d. not given.

4. An infection acquired in the hospital is referred to as a
   a. nosocomial infection.
   b. communal infection.
   c. sustained infection.
   d. antimicrobial infection.

5. Most oral antibiotics should be administered
   a. 1 hr. before meals.
   b. with meals.
   c. 1 hr. after meals.
   d. with a full glass of milk.

6. A condition that occurs when the normal flora is disturbed during antibiotic therapy is known as
   a. organ toxicity.
   b. superinfection.
   c. hypersensitivity.
   d. allergic reaction.

7. Antimycobacterial medication is usually administered in the following way to treat a bacterial infection:
   a. One drug is administered for a period of 7–10 days.
   b. Oral medications are administered for 3–4 weeks.
   c. Two or more antibiotics are used at a time to prevent the development of resistance.
   d. Medications are not administered until the client experiences a temperature above 101°F.

8. When an antibiotic is chosen, the following must be taken into consideration:
   a. Length of time the client has experienced symptoms.
   b. Culture and sensitivity reports.
   c. The client's hydration status.
   d. The client's age.

9. *Objective* symptoms of infection include which of the following?
   a. Lethargy.
   b. Anorexia.
   c. Fever.
   d. Headache.

10. You have just finished instructing your client on measures to help the body fight infections. Which of the following statements by your client would lead you to believe he needs additional instruction?
    a. "I will make sure I get adequate rest."
    b. "I know I must continue to eat and drink lots of fluids."
    c. "I will wash my hands."
    d. "I will take my medicine until I no longer have a fever."

# CHAPTER 34

# Penicillins

## Complete the following sentences

1. Penicillins are the drugs of choice for treating:

     a. _____.

     b. _____.

     c. _____.

     d. _____.

2. Penicillin is used prophylactically for persons who have cardiac problems and are going to undergo _____ or _____.

3. If an infection is caused by staphylococci that is resistant to penicillin G, the following drugs may be effective: _____, _____, _____, _____, and _____.

4. A broad-spectrum, semisynthetic penicillin used for several types of gram-positive and gram-negative bacteria is _____.

5. Ampicillin is effective in treating the following infections: _____, _____, _____, and _____.

6. Unasyn is a combination of _____ and _____.

7. Five penicillins used to treat *Pseudomonas* are: _____, _____, _____, _____, and _____.

8. Prior to administering penicillin, the nurse should ask the client if he or she has ever experienced a _____, _____, _____, or _____ associated with the drug.

9. The trade name for nafcillin is _____, and it is administered _____ in _____ doses _____ mg/kg/day.

10. The route and dosage of the antibiotic depends largely on the _____ of the infection being treated.

11. Probenecid (Benemid) is used concurrently with penicillin to _____ serum drug levels by _____ of penicillin.

12. Penicillin given parenterally is usually given in _____ _____ ml of D5W and infused over _____ minutes.

## Word scramble

Fill in the trade name next to its generic name and circle the trade name in the word find.

1. carbenicillin
   disodium _____.

2. amoxicillin _____.

3. cloxacillin _____.

4. nafcillin _____.

5. ticarcillin _____.

6. azlocillin _____.

7. mazlocillin _____.

8. piperacillin _____.

9. methicillin _____.

10. dicloxacillin _____.

11. oxacillin _____.

12. amoxicillin and potassium clavulinate
    _____.

13. hetacillin _____.

14. amdinocillin _____.

**Word Find**

```
P O R P R O P O X E H E R O E T H L R E R H T E I R B
M R P E N E H P Q A N A N I T V I L E E A N A L I G A
A N O S T H E T I C M O R T I X I L C L X J U P S E R
P I N S W I L M O R P T E G O P E X O P I U S N D A B
S D I I T X W R A N G E R M U T I T A S H E I O D S I
R I T R L A C N O C T R A I L E H E R I E L N A V A S
I R I P I D P I L I W T H E M A R C O V Z R E H P R O
T I C A R L S H D A P Y T O N V E R S A P E N P O R P
E P S U G A J E I E P A R E R P A T I I A H S E D A E
F E R G T I C U L N R A C O A C T I N N G S Y S T D M
R M S M S I C U M U L E N A I D O N E A L C I P I Y E
E I G E O P E N T C I N M O E S T A P H C I L L I N E
C C G N E U A I O R A I L S P O E A S P O T O N P A H
O I L T E A B P N P Y H A Y L P G T A I P E L O R P L
D T A I P R O E O X Y P H E N E O I M O E H T E L E H
E E N N A L E N T W I R E H T H P I P R A C I L C N A
I R A B A R B I T W I O P I A N E P C D I T T R O M L
T E R E T I C U A C T M E Z L I N D I N E H S E D A F
```

## Review questions

1. Your client has had subacute bacterial endocarditis. His physician is likely to recommend
   a. prophylactic use of penicillin prior to visiting the dentist.
   b. low-dose penicillin therapy for the rest of his life.
   c. double the recommended dose of penicillin if he undergoes a surgical procedure.
   d. using only *Pseudomonas*-resistant antibiotics.

2. Penicillin may be the drug of choice for treating which of the following infections?
   a. Syphilis.
   b. Vaginitis.
   c. Acne.
   d. Gastritis and pancreatitis.

3. A broad-spectrum, semisynthetic penicillin used to treat several gram-positive and gram-negative infections is
   a. dicloxacillin (Dynapen).
   b. nafcillin (Unipen).
   c. ampicillin (Omnipen).
   d. methicillin (Staphcillin).

4. A penicillin used to treat *Pseudomonas* is
   a. nafeillin (Unipen).
   b. amoxicillin and potassium clavulinate (Augmentin).
   c. amoxicillin (Amoxil).
   d. ticarcillin (Ticar).

5. Your client weighs 90 lbs. and is to receive 4 doses of Unipen. The total daily dose is 50 mg/kg/day. How much will your client receive per dose?
   a. 250 mg.
   b. 500 mg.
   c. 1000 mg.
   d. 2000 mg.

6. Probenecid (Benemid) is used with penicillin to
   a. increase serum drug levels.
   b. prevent an anaphylactic reaction.
   c. break down the bacteria cell wall.
   d. decrease the amount of penicillin needed for a therapeutic effect.

7. Administration of large doses of penicillin G can produce the following electrolyte disturbance:
   a. Hyponatremia.
   b. Hypocalcemia.
   c. Hyperkalemia.
   d. Hyperchloremia.

8. Common side effects of high-dose antibiotic therapy are
   a. nausea, vomiting, diarrhea.
   b. anorexia and weight loss.
   c. constipation and fluid retention.
   d. syncope, tachycardia, hypotension.

9. Superinfections can be caused by
   a. antibiotic therapy.
   b. exposure to nosocomial infections.
   c. exposure to opportunistic micro-organisms.
   d. resistant micro-organisms.

10. You should contact the physician if the client states that he or she has previously experienced which of the following symptoms after the administration of penicillin?
   a. Nausea, vomiting, diarrhea.
   b. Swelling or difficulty breathing.
   c. Constipation and fluid retention.
   d. Frequency of urination and weight loss.

## Critical thinking case study

Mr. B., a type I diabetic, is admitted to the hospital with severe dehydration. He has recently returned from a trip and has been having diarrhea since he returned home. His stool culture reveals *Shigella* and he is started on ampicillin and sulbactam (Unasyn) IV.

1. Explain why these drugs were chosen for Mr. B.

2. Explain the rationale for the parenteral route of administration.

The following morning, you enter Mr. B.'s room and find that Mr. B. has a dull red rash on his face and chest.

3. Identify and prioritize your nursing activities.

# CHAPTER 35

# Cephalosporins

## Complete the following sentences

1. Cephalosporins inhibit formation of _____.

2. They act against _____ and _____.

3. There are _____, _____, and _____ generation cephalosporins.

4. Cephalosporins are commonly used for

    a. _____    d. _____

    b. _____    e. _____

    c. _____    f. _____

5. Delayed reactions that someone might exhibit after receiving cephalosporins include

    _____, _____, and

    _____.

6. Four first-generation cephalosporins are cephalexin (_____) and cephradine

    (_____), cefazolin (_____), and (_____).

7. An example of a second generation drug is cefaclor (_____.)

8. Third-generation cephalosporins are used to treat infections

    _____ and in clients who are

    _____.

9. Two examples of a third-generation cephalosporin are cefotetan (_____) and ceftriax-
    one (_____).

10. The maximum daily dose of cefotetan in a life-threatening infection is _____ grams. One problem
    that can occur with this dosage is _____. Rocephin can be administered
    _____ time(s) a day.

11. In _____, all cephalosporins except for Cefobid should be reduced by _____ %.

12. Nephrotoxicity from cephalosporin administration is exhibited by _____,
    _____, and _____.

13. Cefamandole (_____), cefoperazone (_____), and moxalactan
    (_____) may cause bleeding because they

    _____.

14. When _____ are administered with a cephalosporin, there is
    increased incidence of _____.

15. Clients should report the occurrence of _____.

# Crossword puzzle

### Across

1. A patient with an anaphylactic reaction to _____ may be sensitive to cephalosporins as well.
8. Cephalosporins may aggravate _____ impairment.
9. Third-generation cephalosporins can penetrate into _____ fluid and aid meningeal infections.
10. Preferred for intramuscular administration.
11. Especially active against *B. fragilis.*

### Down

2. The first third-generation cephalosporin approved for one daily dosage.
3. This drug causes severe intestinal bleeding and is no longer recommended for use.
4. First-generation cephalosporins are often used to prevent infections after _____ surgery.
5. These drugs decrease the effects of cephalosporins.
6. This drug is excreted in bile and its half-life is prolonged in hepatic failure.
7. The first oral cephalosporin, still extensively used.

# Review questions

1. A delayed reaction that someone might exhibit after receiving a cephalosporin is
   a. hypertension.
   b. bradycardia.
   c. drug fever.
   d. gingivitis.

2. Which of the following drugs are recommended for serious infections?
   a. First-generation cephalosporins.
   b. Second-generation cephalosporins.
   c. Third-generation cephalosporins.
   d. All of the above.

3. Cephalosporins are commonly used for
   a. bacterial endocarditis.
   b. oral *Candida albicans* infection.
   c. gastritis.
   d. surgical prophylaxis.

4. Third generation cephalosporins are used to treat infections in persons who
   a. are immunosuppressed.
   b. have a cardiac history of cardiac disorders.
   c. have renal failure.
   d. are allergic to penicillin.

5. The physician orders Rocephin 2 gm in 100 ml over 45 minutes. How fast will you run the IV per minute (using macro gtt. tubing 10 drops = 1 cc)?
   a. 12 drops per minute.
   b. 22 drops per minute.
   c. 32 drops per minute.
   d. 42 drops per minute.

6. When administering large doses of cephalosporins IV, the nurse needs to observe for
   a. tachycardia.
   b. septicemia.
   c. thrombophlebitis.
   d. hypertension.

7. In renal failure, the dosage of cephalosporins should be
   a. increased.
   b. decreased.
   c. withheld.
   d. administered with a second antibiotic.

8. A client experiencing nephrotoxicity secondary to cephalosporin administration may exhibit
   a. an elevated pulse.
   b. an elevated sodium.
   c. blood in the urine.
   d. casts in the urine.

9. Certain cephalosporins can cause bleeding because they
   a. decrease the platelet count.
   b. kill bacteria that produce vitamin K.
   c. inhibit absorption of clotting factors.
   d. increase the excretion of vitamin K.

10. Clients may experience renal toxicity when cephalosporins are administered with
    a. anticoagulants.
    b. penicillins.
    c. probenecid (Benemid).
    d. loop diuretics.

## Critical thinking case study

B.J., a 6-year-old, is admitted for treatment of Haemophilus influenza infection. Her physician orders penicillin G. After her initial treatment, B.J. develops nausea, vomiting, and hypotension. (The learner may need to use additional sources to answer the questions.)

1. Identify and prioritize your nursing actions.

B.J.'s physician changes her medication to cephalonthin (Keflin). B.J.'s mother is extremely anxious about starting a new medication.

2. Discuss the rationale for changing the medication with B.J.'s mother and identify why this drug is an appropriate alternative to penicillin.

3. Identify what you will be assessing for when you initially administer the medication.

4. Identify what will be included in an ongoing assessment of B.J.

# CHAPTER 36

# Aminoglycosides

## Complete the following sentences

1. Aminoglycosides are used to treat infections caused by _____ microorganisms.

2. Aminoglycosides are used intravenously to treat _____.

3. They are also used orally to _____ which produces _____.

4. Aminoglycosides are _____ and _____ and must be administered cautiously in the presence of _____.

5. Amikacin is used to treat infections _____.
   The dosage is _____/kg/day

6. If a client weighs 120 lbs and she is to receive the Amikacin in 3 equal doses, how many milligrams will she receive per dose? _____.

7. Neomycin is recommended for _____ or _____ use only. Neomycin is used to treat infections of the _____, _____, and _____.

8. Before administering aminoglycosides, the nurse should
   a. _____.
   b. _____.
   c. analyze medications, assess other drugs _____.
   d. _____.

9. While your client is receiving aminoglycosides,
   a. monitor _____ and _____.
   b. force fluids to _____.

10. Peak levels should be obtained _____ minutes after a dose. Both peak and _____ levels are necessary to establish a therapeutic serum level. Trough levels are taken 30–60 minutes before the next dose. For gentamicin and tobramycin, peak levels of _____ mg/ml and trough levels of _____mg/ml have been associated with nephrotoxicity.

11. When administering aminoglycosides, avoid concurrent administration with _____.

12. Aminoglycosides should be given no longer than _____ days.

## Review questions

1. When administering aminoglycosides, the nurse should observe for the following symptoms associated with ototoxicity:

   a. Tinnitus and ataxia.

   b. Double vision.

   c. Pain and swelling of ear canal.

   d. Nausea and vomiting.

2. Aminoglycosides are used orally to treat

   a. hepatic failure.

   b. renal failure.

   c. respiratory infections.

   d. skin infection.

3. The physician orders gentamicin for a child weighing 44 lbs. If the dose range is 6–7.5 mg/kg/day, and the child is to receive the medication t.i.d., how many milligrams should the child receive per dose?

   a. 20 mg.

   b. 40 mg.

   c. 60 mg.

   d. 80 mg.

4. Peak serum drug levels for gentamicin should be drawn

   a. 15 minutes after a dose.

   b. 30 minutes after a dose.

   c. 2 hours after a dose.

   d. 4 hours after a dose.

5. While your client is receiving aminoglycosides, you should monitor

   a. liver function studies.

   b. intake and output.

   c. apical pulse.

   d. skin color.

6. When administering aminoglycosides, avoid concurrent administration of

   a. penicillins.

   b. beta blockers.

   c. calcium channel blockers.

   d. diuretics.

7. If neomycin is used before bowel surgery to suppress intestinal flora, this may

   a. eliminate the need for antibiotics in the postoperative period.

   b. decrease the possibility of infections that can occur following surgery.

   c. reduce the number of antibiotics prescribed during the preoperative period.

   d. enhance healing.

8. Aminoglycosides can be nephrotoxic. The most sensitive indicator of compromised renal function is

   a. increased blood pressure.

   b. weight gain.

   c. a decrease in urinary output.

   d. increased serum creatinine.

9. For which of the following would a person receiving oral aminoglycosides be at high risk?

   a. Injury secondary to confusion.

   b. Decreased cardiac output.

   c. Altered bowel elimination.

   d. Injury secondary to bleeding.

10. Which of the following statements is *true* regarding aminoglycoside antibiotics?

   a. Gram-negative microorganisms are resistant to aminoglycoside therapy.

   b. Aminoglycosides cannot be used in conjunction with any other antibiotic.

   c. The recommended length of administration is no longer than 10 days.

   d. Aminoglycosides break down the bacterial cell wall.

## Critical thinking case study

Mrs. J. is being treated with tobramycin (Nebcin) for a pseudomonas infection.

1. Identify the assessments that will be done before and during treatment with this drug.

Mrs. J.'s urinary output begins to drop.

2. Identify your nursing actions.

You speak to the physician on call about Mrs. J.'s decreased urinary output. He orders furosemide (Lasix) 80 mg IV push.

3. Discuss what you will do next.

# CHAPTER 37

# Tetracyclines

## Complete the following sentences

1. Tetracycline is effective against _____ and _____ organisms as well

   as _____, _____, and some _____

   _____.

2. Tetracycline decreases the effectiveness of _____ and _____.

3. Tetracycline is used for

   a. _____.

   b. _____.

   c. _____.

   d. _____.

   e. _____.

   f. _____.

   g. _____.

4. Tetracycline is contraindicated for persons who _____, are

   _____, or who are pregnant.

5. If tetracyline is administered to children, it can cause _____ and

   _____.

6. Oral tetracycline preparations should be administered _____.

7. Tetracyclines should not be administered with _____.

8. When taking a tetracycline you should avoid exposure to _____ because it may cause

   _____ _____.

9. _____ is more likely to occur with tetracycline than with other antibiotics.

10. Liver toxicity produced by tetracyclines may occur if the person has _____

    or is _____.

11. Two drugs that increase the effects of tetracycline include _____ and

    _____ .

12. Phenytoin (Dilantin) will _____ the effects of tetracyclines.

13. Persons taking tetracyclines should report the following side effects to the physician:

    _____, _____, _____, _____, _____ itching.

14. Do not take _____ products with tetracyclines because they will produce nonabsorbable

    compounds.

## Review questions

1.  You know your health teaching has been effective if your client who is taking a tetracycline states that she should
    a.  take the drug with milk.
    b.  contact the physician if she develops acne.
    c.  take it only if she is going to be inside all day.
    d.  avoid taking the drug if she becomes pregnant.

2.  Tetracyclines can be detrimental if given to persons between the ages of
    a.  1 and 8 years.
    b.  9 and 16 years.
    c.  60 and 69 years.
    d.  70 and 79 years.

3.  A tetracycline is prescribed for Mrs. P. What information should you give to Mrs. P.?
    a.  "Since depression of bone growth occurs, you must take this drug for no more than 1 week."
    b.  "If you become constipated, call us immediately."
    c.  "Avoid direct exposure to the sun."
    d.  "You must drink 8 glasses of water daily when you take this drug."

4.  Mrs. C. tells you that she feels nauseated shortly after taking a tetracycline. What should your recommendations be?
    a.  Take the drug with milk.
    b.  Consume as little water as possible when swallowing the capsule.
    c.  Take 2 tablespoons of Maalox 15 minutes before taking the tetracycline.
    d.  Take the drug with food, but avoid milk and milk products.

5.  Mrs. A. is taking a tetracycline to treat her acne. Which statement would lead you to believe that she needs further teaching?
    a.  "I will take my iron and the tetracycline at different times."
    b.  "If I experience diarrhea or a skin rash, I will contact my physician."
    c.  "If I lie out in the sun for short periods, it will help clean up my acne."
    d.  "I will take the medication an hour before meals."

6.  Mr. J. was treated with an erythromycin for pneumonia. When he returned to the office, he still had chest congestion so his physician ordered a tetracycline. Your instructions to Mr. J. should include:
    a.  "Take the tetracycline until your symptoms subside."
    b.  "Make sure you finish the medication from the previous prescription."
    c.  "Take the tetracycline until you have finished the prescription."
    d.  "Restrict your fluids and monitor your urinary output."

7.  When you are caring for a client taking a tetracycline, you should assess him or her for the following adverse effects:
    a.  Headache.
    b.  Diarrhea.
    c.  Weight gain.
    d.  Blurred vision.

8.  Which drug, if administered with a tetracycline, could modify its actions?
    a.  Antacids.
    b.  Antihypertensives.
    c.  Anticholinergics.
    d.  Antidepressants.

9.  Miss A., an 18-year-old who is taking a tetracycline for acne, should be instructed to discontinue the medication if
    a.  she develops constipation.
    b.  her stomach is upset when she takes the medication.
    c.  her acne improves.
    d.  she develops a skin rash.

10.  Tetracyclines are eliminated primarily by
    a.  renal excretion.
    b.  liver metabolism.
    c.  gastrointestinal enzymes.
    d.  biliary metabolism.

## Critical thinking case study

M.J., a 16-year-old high school student, comes to the dermatologist to be treated for acne. She is given a prescription for a tetracycline.

1.  Identify the assessments that will be done before she starts the medication.

2.  Discuss the instructions you will give M.J. before she starts the medication.

M.J. returns to the office in 4 weeks and states that the medication has been ineffective.

3.  Identify the information you will elicit from M.J. to help make your assessment.

After additional instructions, M.J. decides to continue the medication. She returns to the office 4 weeks later, complaining of a sore throat.

4.  Identify your nursing actions.

# CHAPTER 38

# Macrolides

## Complete the following sentences

1. Erythromycin is _____ rather than bactericidal except in _____ doses.

2. Clinical indications for using erythromycin include

   a. _____.

   b. _____.

   c. _____.

   d. _____.

   e. _____.

   f. _____.

3. Erythromycin is contraindicated or must be used with caution in clients who

   _____.

4. Macrolides are primarily effective against _____.

5. Clarithromycin must be reduced in clients with _____.

6. Erythromycin is used with neomycin preoperatively to _____.

7. Oral azithromycin should be administered _____.

8. Erythromycin should be administered on _____ stomach.

9. Common side effects of erythromycin are _____ and _____.

10. Symptoms of hepatotoxicity include _____.

## True or false

_____ 1. Erythromycin is used as a substitute for penicillin.

_____ 2. In renal failure, the dosage of erythromycin needs to be reduced.

_____ 3. If an aminoglycoside is administered with erythromycin, it will decrease the effect of the erythromycin.

_____ 4. It is common for anaphylactic reactions to occur as a result of the administration of erythromycin.

_____ 5. Erythromycin is the drug of choice for meningitis.

## Review questions

1. Erythromycin is the drug of choice for treating:
   a. Legionnaire's disease.
   b. bacterial endocarditis.
   c. urinary tract infections.
   d. acne.

2. Erythromycin is used with neomycin to
   a. prevent whooping cough.
   b. suppress intestinal bacteria.
   c. eliminate diphtheria.
   d. treat diarrhea.

3. Erythromycin should be administered
   a. with meals.
   b. on an empty stomach.
   c. with milk an hour before meals.
   d. with crackers and no fluids to prevent nausea.

4. Macrolides must be used with caution in clients who have
   a. renal disease.
   b. liver disease.
   c. diabetes mellitus.
   d. hypertension.

5. Which of the following medications, if administered with erythromycin, will increase the effect of the erythromycin?
   a. Penicillins.
   b. Tetracyclines.
   c. Ampicillin.
   d. Chloramphenical (Chloromycetin).

6. The following medication may increase the effects of erythromycin when the two drugs are administered together:
   a. Furosemide (Lasix)
   b. Aspirin.
   c. Vitamin E.
   d. Aminoglycosides.

7. A common side effect that occurs after the administration of erythromycin is
   a. anaphylaxis.
   b. urticaria.
   c. nausea.
   d. colitis.

8. Which of the following medications, if administered concurrently with erythromycin, will decrease its effects?
   a. Antacids.
   b. Beta adrenergic blockers.
   c. Calcium channel blockers.
   d. Antidepressants.

9. Erythromycin can be used as a substitute for penicillin to treat
   a. meningitis.
   b. botulism.
   c. chlamydial infection.
   d. syphilis.

10. M.J., who weighs 44 lbs., is being treated with erythromycin ethylsuccinate (EES) for pneumonia. The recommended dose is 30 mg/kg/day. The medication is to be administered q6h. How much medication should M.J. receive per dose?
    a. 100 mg.
    b. 125 mg.
    c. 150 mg.
    d. 175 mg

## Critical thinking case study

Mr. R., a 40-year-old attorney, has been experiencing chills, fever, and lethargy for 2 days. He is seen by his physician in the office, diagnosed with pneumonia, and started on erythromycin.

1.  Identify the initial assessments that the physician would have done to establish his diagnosis.

2.  Identify the instructions that you will give Mr. R. before he returns home.

Mrs. R. calls you the next day to tell you that her husband has been vomiting on and off since he started the medication.

3.  Specify what your instruction to Mrs. R. will be.

Mr. R. is admitted to the hospital and started on erythromycin IV. He continues to vomit.

4.  Identify what you will do.

# CHAPTER 39

# Miscellaneous Anti-infectives

## Complete the following sentences

1. Aztreonam (_____) is effective against a wide spectrum of _____ bacteria.

2. The advantage of Aztreonam (_____) over other antimicrobial agents is that it:

   a. _____

   b. _____

3. The indication for the use of imipenem/cilastatin (_____) is for the treatment of

   _____.

4. Norfloxacin (_____) is indicated for _____.

5. Ciprofloxacin (_____) is effective against

   _____.

6. Chloramphenicol (_____) is the drug of choice for treating

   _____ and is also used for _____.

7. Colistin (_____) is used topically for _____. Colistin in an otic

   suspension is administered for _____.

8. Spectinomycin (_____) is used to treat _____ in

   persons who are allergic to penicillin.

9. _____ (Vancocin) is only used for _____ infections because it is

   _____ and ototoxic.

10. In the presence of renal impairment, the dosage of the following drugs needs to be reduced:

    a. _____.

    b. _____.

    c. _____.

## Review questions

1. The nurse will monitor the following lab values for Mr. O. who is taking chloramphenicol (Chloromycetin):

   a. Blood sugar.                          c. Potassium level.
   b. Platelet count.                       d. Calcium level.

2. When teaching Mrs. C. about vancomycin (Vancocin), the nurse should include the following information: "We will be monitoring your

   a. blood sugars."                        c. kidney function."
   b. liver function."                      d. RBC."

3. After the third dose of vancomycin (Vancocin), Mrs. H. is to have a serum level drawn. Which of the following would indicate a therapeutic level of vancomycin (Vancocin)?

   a. 1.5–2.5 µg/ml.
   b. 3.5–8.5 µg/ml.

   c. 10–25 µg/ml.
   d. 35–55 µg/ml.

4. Which of the following nursing diagnoses apply to Mr. C. who is receiving chloramphenicol (Chloromycetin)?

   a. Fluid volume deficit.
   b. High risk for alteration in nutrition.

   c. Decreased cardiac output.
   d. High risk for injury; bleeding.

5. Miss C. has developed pseudomembranous colitis secondary to the administration of antibiotics. The drug most effective in the oral treatment of colitis is

   a. vancomycin (Vancocin).
   b. polymyxin B (Aerosporin).

   c. norfloxacin (Noroxin).
   d. ciprofloxacin (Cipro).

6. The nurse should monitor clients receiving aztreonam (Azactam) for potential side effects which include

   a. superinfection.
   b. liver toxicity.

   c. renal toxicity.
   d. gastrointestinal bleeding.

7. Which of the following antibiotics preserves the body's anaerobic flora?

   a. Aztreonam (Azactam).
   b. Ciprofloxacin (Cipro).

   c. Colistin (Coly-Mycin).
   d. Chloramphenicol (Chloromycetin).

8. The drug of choice for treatment of gonococcal infections resistant to penicillin is

   a. ciprofloxacin (Cipro).
   b. chloramphenicol (Chloromycetin).

   c. spectinomycin (Trobicin).
   d. vancomycin (Vancocin).

9. Drugs administered concurrently with vancomycin (Vancocin) that increase the effects of vancomycin include:

   a. ciprofloxacin (Cipro) and bacitracin.
   b. chloramphenicol (Chloromycetin) and neomycin.

   c. imipenem/cilastatin and neomycin.
   d. amphotericin B (Fungizone) and cisplatin (Platinol).

10. Which of the following statements by your client, who is receiving imipenem/cilastatin (Primaxin) leads you to believe that she has understood the teaching that you have done?

    a. "Nausea, vomiting, and diarrhea are common side effects of this medication."
    b. "I need to drink plenty of fluids and weigh myself daily."

    c. "I will not worry if I see blood in my urine; I know that is a common side effect."
    d. "I will take the medication when I am sitting down because I know dizziness is common."

## Critical thinking case study

Mr. H. is admitted with a temperature of 104°F, chills, nausea, and vomiting. He is diagnosed with pneumonia. Blood cultures are drawn and he is started on aztreonam (Azactam).

1. Identify your nursing actions.

Mr. H. continues to have a fever despite the administration of fluids and IV antibiotics. The results of the blood culture reveal that Mr. H. has a severe infection caused by penicillin-resistant staphylococci. Vancomycin (Vancocin) is ordered.

2. Explain why the physician changed Mr. H.'s medication.

3. Identify the nursing implications of the administration of vancomycin (Vancocin).

# CHAPTER 40

# Sulfonamides and Urinary Antiseptics

## Complete the following sentences

1. Sulfonamides are useful in urinary tract infections caused by _____, _____, or _____.

2. Topical sulfonamides are useful in prevention and treatment of _____, _____, _____, and other _____.

3. Sulfonamides are contraindicated in persons _____, _____, _____, _____, _____, and persons allergic to _____.

4. Cinoxacin (_____) is used for the treatment of initial and recurrent UTIs. It is most effective against _____ bacteria.

5. Methenamine mandelate (_____) and methenamine hippurate (_____) are used for _____ of urine. _____ may be administered with these drugs to acidify the urine.

6. Nitrofurantoin (_____, _____) is effective against _____ and _____ organisms.

7. Phenazopyridine (_____) relieves _____, _____, _____, and _____. It turns the urine _____.

8. When a person is experiencing a UTI, he or she should force fluids to produce a urinary output of _____ cc a day.

9. With sulfonamide therapy the urine pH should be _____.

10. With mandelamine therapy, urine pH must be _____.

11. In older adults using combination drugs, sulfamethoxazole and trimethoprim (_____) and (_____), they are at risk for developing _____, _____, and _____.

## True or false

_____ 1. When taking urinary tract antiseptics, you should drink 1200–1500 cc/day.

_____ 2. Persons taking nitrofurantoin (Macrodantin) should not take antacids.

_____ 3. Tetracyclines should not be used with sulfonamides because it increases their effects.

_____ 4. If a skin rash appears after sulfonamide therapy begins, the dosage should be decreased.

_____ 5. Sulfonamides suppress bacterial growth by interfering with microorganisms required to produce folic acid.

## Review questions

1. Your health teaching for methenamine mandelate (Mandelamine) would include the following.
   a. "Take ascorbic acid with the medication to acidify the urine."
   b. "Take sodium bicarbonate with the medication to make the urine alkaline."
   c. "Limit your fluid intake to 1500 cc/day."
   d. "While you are taking this drug limit your intake of food high in sodium."

2. Phenazopyridine (Pyridium) is a urinary tract analgesic used to relieve which of the following symptoms?
   a. Urinary retention.
   b. Hematuria.
   c. Urgency.
   d. Hesitancy.

3. You will assess Mr. P. who has been started on sulfisoxazole (Gantrisin) for the following adverse effects which may necessitate discontinuation of the drug:
   a. Fever.
   b. Tachycardia.
   c. Elevated blood sugar.
   d. Skin rash.

4. Which of the following statements by Mr. P. leads you to believe that he understands the health teaching you have done about nitrofurantoin (Macrodantin)?
   a. "I know that it will turn my urine orange."
   b. "I will take vitamin C along with the medication."
   c. "I will take the medicine with meals."
   d. "I will take the medicine on an empty stomach."

5. Sulfonamides are used in persons with urinary tract infections to suppress bacterial growth by
   a. interfering with folic acid synthesis.
   b. promoting bacterial replication of DNA.
   c. killing mature, fully formed bacteria.
   d. causing the formation of derivatives of folic acid.

6. Mr. C. is started on trimethoprim (Proloprim) for a urinary tract infection. Prior to administering this drug, the nurse should assess the client for
   a. anemia.
   b. hypertension.
   c. diabetes mellitus.
   d. respiratory failure.

7. Mr. C. has just been started on sulfasalazine (Azulfidine) for ulcerative colitis. Mr. C. is also taking phenytoin (Dilantin) for control of epilepsy. The nurse will monitor Mr. C. for potential drug interactions that could result in
   a. increased toxicity of sulfonamides.
   b. decreased therapeutic effectiveness of sulfonamides.
   c. decreased renal clearance; therefore, increased potential for renal toxicity.
   d. increased risk of hepatotoxicity.

8. Mr. J., a 79-year-old male, is started on sulfamethoxazole-trimethoprim (Bactrim) for urinary tract infection; he should be observed for adverse effects which include
   a. liver toxicity.
   b. renal failure.
   c. bone marrow depression.
   d. congestive heart failure.

9. A person receiving phenazopyridine (Pyridium) should be informed that it will change the color of urine to
   a. bluish-green.
   b. reddish-orange.
   c. brown.
   d. black.

10. A measure that the nurse can encourage clients to use to reduce the risk of recurrent urinary tract infections is to
    a. increase alkaline foods in the diet.
    b. take tub baths, soaking 15 minutes daily.
    c. use sterile gauze pads to cleanse after urinating.
    d. force fluids to 3000 cc daily.

## Critical thinking case study

M. has had type I diabetes mellitus for 10 years and is poorly controlled. She is being seen today for a urinary tract infection (UTI). She has had 12 UTIs in 10 years. Her physician has ordered sulfamethoxazole-trimethoprim (Bactrim).

1. Develop a teaching plan that will address her current diagnosis as well as encourage compliance with her diabetes treatment plan.

2. Identify ways of fostering compliance.

3. Discuss with M. ways of preventing future UTIs.

# CHAPTER 41

# Antitubercular Drugs

## Complete the following sentences

1. Today, the recommended length of initial treatment for TB is _____ months.

2. The primary drugs used for initial treatment are _____, _____, _____, and _____.

3. Secondary drugs are used when _____.

4. An indication for prophylactic use of INH would be a positive _____.

5. INH should not be given to persons _____ who have had a reaction _____ or _____.

6. Before a person receives rifampin he or she should be told that it may turn _____ a _____ color.

7. The dosage of ethambutol is calculated according to _____.

8. The four drugs used for secondary treatment of TB include _____, _____, _____, and _____.

9. When INH is being administered to an older adult, _____ should be monitored regularly.

10. To minimize nausea, vomiting, and diarrhea, PAS and ethionamide are given _____.

11. Rifampin should be administered _____ a meal.

12. An elevated AST or ALT would indicate _____.

13. An elevated BUN and creatinine would indicate _____.

14. The following reactions should be reported to the physician:
    a. _____.
    b. _____.
    c. _____.
    d. _____.
    e. _____.

15. Early symptoms of hypersensitivity to antitubercular drugs are _____, _____, and _____ and are likely to occur between the _____ and _____ weeks of drug therapy.

## Review questions

1. Your client who is taking INH (Laniazid), rifampin (Rifadin), and pyrazinamide calls you because her urine is reddish-orange. You tell her:

   a. "You may be bleeding so you should see your doctor immediately."

   b. "This may be due to hepatic toxicity. You should discontinue the drugs."

   c. "You have a urinary tract infection; drink plenty of fluids."

   d. "This is a normal response to rifampin."

2. Prior to initiating INH therapy, you should ask your client the following question:

   a. "Are you pregnant?"

   b. "Are you allergic to aspirin?"

   c. "Do you have a family history of diabetes?"

   d. "Have you ever been hypertensive?"

3. Your client appears to have yellow sclera. What other findings would lead you to believe that she may be experiencing hepatic toxicity from the antitubercular drugs?

   a. Diarrhea.

   b. Numbness and tingling.

   c. Visual changes.

   d. Clay-colored stools.

4. Which of the following drugs should be taken with food to prevent nausea, vomiting, and diarrhea?

   a. Rifampin (Rifadin).

   b. Para-amino salicylic acid (PAS).

   c. INH (Laniazid).

   d. Streptomycin.

5. Your client is receiving antitubercular drug therapy. You notice that her urinary output has dropped in the past week. Which lab values should you check before you administer her next dose?

   a. Hematocrit and hemoglobin.

   b. BUN and creatinine.

   c. AST and ALT.

   d. Urine culture and sensitivity.

6. Early symptoms of a hypersensitivity reaction to antitubercular drugs are

   a. nausea and diarrhea.

   b. bradycardia and hypertension.

   c. fever and tachycardia.

   d. bleeding gums.

7. Your client who weighs 200 lbs. is to receive 1500 mg ethambutol daily. If the recommended dose is 15/mg/kg daily, this dose is

   a. low.

   b. high.

   c. appropriate.

8. You should begin to see the therapeutic effects of antitubercular drug therapy in

   a. 5–7 days.

   b. 7–10 days.

   c. 2–3 weeks.

   d. 6 weeks.

9. You will know that your client with tuberculosis is improving as the result of drug therapy when his

   a. weight decreases.

   b. tidal volume increases.

   c. sputum decreases.

   d. skin test improves.

10. The recommended length of initial treatment for someone who has been exposed but has a negative tuberculin test is

    a. 10 days.

    b. 3 months.

    c. 6 months.

    d. 12 months.

## Critical thinking case study

Miss G. is a 25-year-old public health nurse who has a positive PPD test but a negative chest x-ray for tuberculosis. She is started on INH.

1.  Identify what your instruction will be for Miss G.

Miss G. calls your office 6 months after starting the medication and states that she has stopped menstruating and that the skin has a yellow cast.

2.  Identify your response.

# CHAPTER 42

# Antiviral Drugs

## True or false

_____ 1. Viruses can live for hours outside of a living organism.

_____ 2. Acyclovir (Zovirax) inactivates the herpes virus and prevents recurrence of the disease.

_____ 3. Amantadine (Symmetrel) may be useful in the treatment of influenza A infections.

_____ 4. Ganciclovir (Cytovene) is effective in treating the systemic symptoms associated with herpes.

_____ 5. Ribavirin (Virazole) is administered by inhalation for the treatment of respiratory syncytial virus (RSV).

_____ 6. Zidovudine (Retrovir) is the current drug of choice for treating AIDS.

_____ 7. Live attenuated viral vaccines are potentially toxic and should only be used on an experimental basis.

_____ 8. Ophthalmic antiviral preparations can cause inflammation of the eyelids.

_____ 9. Persons who have visible herpes lesions will not spread the disease if they apply acyclovir before having sexual intercourse.

_____ 10. There are many vaccines available that will prevent viral diseases including poliomyelitis, mumps, yellow fever, and rabies.

_____ 11. Zidovudine (Retrovir) is used for persons with AIDS to prevent the occurrence of opportunistic infections.

_____ 12. Viral infections can occur without any signs and symptoms of illness.

_____ 13. Repeated courses of acyclovir (Zovirax) therapy may result in the emergence of acyclovir-resistant viral strains.

_____ 14. When antipyretics and anti-inflammatory drugs are administered with zidovudine (Retrovir), there will be an increased risk of adverse effects.

_____ 15. Insomnia and ataxia are adverse effects associated with the use of amantadine (Symmetrel).

## Review questions

1. Adverse effects of ganciclovir (Cytovene) that the nurse needs to assess for include
   a. stomatitis.
   b. hypertension.
   c. arrhythmias.
   d. thrombocytopenia.

2. Mr. J. has herpes simplex encephalitis. An expected outcome after the administration of vidarabine (Vira-A) is
   a. decreased fever.
   b. decreased heart rate.
   c. increased blood pressure.
   d. increased respiratory rate.

3. Live attenuated viral vaccines should not be administered to persons who are
   a. diabetic.
   b. pregnant.
   c. under age 2.
   d. over age 70.

4. Mr. J. is ordered trifluridine (Viroptic) for treatment of recurrent epithelial keratitis. Which of the following statements by Mr. J. leads you to believe that he understands how to use the medication?

   a. "After I take this medication, I may notice tearing and nasal congestion."
   b. "After I administer the medication, I will apply cold compresses to my eyes."

   c. "I should use this drug for no longer than 3 weeks."
   d. "I will use the medication in the morning and before I go to bed."

5. Mr. J., a 21-year-old male, is being started on zidovudine (Retrovir) for treatment of AIDS. Which of the following statements by Mr. J. leads you to believe that he understands the teaching that you have done?

   a. "Zidovudine (Retrovir) inactivates the virus and prevents recurrence of the disease."
   b. "Zidovudine (Retrovir) therapy may result in the development of zidoxudine (Retrovir)-resistant viral strains.

   c. "Zidovudine (Retrovir) slows the progression of the disease but does not cure it."
   d. "Zidovudine (Retrovir) prevents the occurrence of opportunistic infections."

6. Infants who are being treated with ribavirin (Virazole) for RSV should be assessed for

   a. hepatotoxicity.
   b. renal failure.

   c. ventricular tachycardia.
   d. deteriorating pulmonary function.

7. Which of the following instructions should you give to Mrs. B. who is taking trifluridine (Viroptic) for an eye infection?

   a. "Use sterile gloves when you are applying the ointment."
   b. "Initially, you should administer the drops every 2 hours while you are awake."

   c. "The medication may temporarily cause yellowing of the sclera."
   d. "The crystals should be dissolved in water and you should use an eye cup to apply the solution to the eye."

8. The use of amantadine (Symmetrel) for treatment of influenza A is recommended for use in

   a. all adults.
   b. persons with a family history of heart disease.

   c. persons with chronic lung disease.
   d. children under the age of 2.

9. You are to administer acyclovir (Zovirax) intravenously. The recommended dose is 5 mg/kg q8h. Your client weighs 132 lbs. How much medication will you administer per dose?

   a. 100 mg.
   b. 200 mg.

   c. 300 mg.
   d. 400 mg.

10. Which of the following medications, if administered concurrently with zidovudine (Retrovir), will alter its effects?

    a. Anticholinergics.
    b. Cholinergics.

    c. acetaminophen (Tylenol).
    d. Maalox.

## Critical thinking case study

JJ, a 32-year-old male, has recently been diagnosed with HIV and is started on zidovudine (Retrovir).

1. Discuss the instructions that you will give him.

2. Identify three nursing diagnoses that would be appropriate for JJ.

JJ's disease progresses rapidly. Within 3 years, he develops AIDS and has contracted several opportunistic infections. He is presently being seen for cytomegalovirus retinitis for which the doctor orders ganciclovir (Cytovene).

3. Discuss the instructions that you will give him.

JJ calls you because he has noticed some bleeding. He is crying on the phone and states, "I don't want to die."

4. Discuss how you will respond to JJ.

# CHAPTER 43

# Antifungal Drugs

## Matching exercise: terms and concepts

_____ 1. Tinea pedis.

_____ 2. A highly contagious fungal infection spread by sharing towels and hair brushes.

_____ 3. Thrush.

_____ 4. This can occur as a result of the administration of antibodies.

_____ 5. Found in soil and organic debris.

_____ 6. Causes a respiratory infection that resembles pneumonia or tuberculosis.

_____ 7. Used to treat fungal infections of the eye.

_____ 8. Drug used to treat athlete's foot.

_____ 9. Drug used to treat blastomycosis.

_____ 10. Drug administered intravenously to treat systemic mycoses.

_____ 11. Adverse effects of this drug include nausea, vomiting, pruritus, and abdominal pain.

_____ 12. Serious adverse effects resulting from the administration of this drug include mental confusion and blood dyscrasias.

_____ 13. The length of time antifungal drugs are administered for.

_____ 14. Signs and symptoms of histoplasmosis, coccidioidomycosis, and blastomycosis.

_____ 15. A drug used for the treatment of tinea versicolor.

A. Athlete's foot.

B. Amphotericin B (Fungizone).

C. Blastomycosis.

D. Miconazole (Monistat).

E. Haloprogin (Halotex).

F. Oral candidiasis.

G. Tinea capitis.

H. Natamycin (Natacyn).

I. Histoplasmosis.

J. Systemic candidiasis.

K. Griseofulvin (Fulvicin).

L. 7–10 days.

M. 2–6 weeks.

N. Cough, fever, malaise.

O. Ketoconazole (Nizoral).

P. Vaginal discharge, burning, itching.

Q. Acrisorcin (Akrinol).

## Word scramble

Fill in the trade name next to the generic name and circle the trade name in the word find.

1. griseofulvin _____.
2. flucytosine _____.
3. econazole _____.
4. zinc undecylenate _____.
5. tolnaftate _____.
6. nystatin _____.

7. natamycin _____.
8. miconazole _____.
9. ketoconazole _____.
10. clotrimazole _____.
11. ciclopirox _____.
12. acrisorcin _____.

**Word Find**

```
D A R D R S C O P B U T A N T I A A D M P H E T N
T E A D A E I O A N T I P A R A I C G R A N T I I
A H S P E C T A Z O L E H Y P S S Y M P A M I N C
C R A E R O D N A A D R E N E P I A S I S M B A T
D X T I N A C T I N R P I N E F N A G R E N E N A
C I G A R E P P Y S O I M I M O N I S T A T M P E
N L O P R O X A M M E A N I T I N A R E V O L A P
D I A T L E V O P H E D D N C G I D N E A R D A H
N E D E D O N I A N T I A I L E A I E D E P E N I
S A R I N U B A T A C I V R E N I L O H C I T N A
I I A A B O S A H I S L P N I N E R S S T I T D U
I M M A D S U M O Y U E I I I P E O T N C I G R T
P N S N I I D I M F E R P P I N S R I C A I C A O
N E I T M S A P I C H E C E O P E C G D A I B C A
S Y M C H A A T M P P H E L O T R I M I N E S I U
E L N C O T E P E C O T I I T O L I Y E C Y C B T
I N E I H T O N T L V I N P T I A N C H O C M E O
A L I E Z I I N I E E E H O G A D R O N B L I N N
P E T P E O H N C R L A G R N R O G S C O T D I O
N I A H E P R D E P H R N T E C N U T A N T R I M
C R N R A R P A K R I N O L I C N T A I T A I S I
T A O E G A N G L I A D E N A M A A T O S I A H C
T N A I S C O P O L A M I N E P N B I A M O S O M
N T C W P H E D R I A S N A T A C Y N R E N I M A
A I I H A P P R I O D L N I I F I R T A S I S M N
N C T P O P H I A S R D E S F A E P I N E P I N E
I C I G R E N I L O H C I T N A P H E D R E I S T
```

## Review questions

1. The drug most commonly used to treat *Candida albicans* is
   a. acrisorcin (Akrinol).
   b. tolnaftate (Tinactin).
   c. griseofulvin (Fulvicin).
   d. nystatin (Mycostatin).

2. Which of the following medications, if administered concurrently with ketoconazole (Nizoral), will decrease its effect?
   a. Diuretics.
   b. Steroids.
   c. Antacids.
   d. Antibiotics.

3. Mrs. G., who weighs 90 lbs., is to receive griseofulvin (Fulvicin) 10 mg/kg daily. If Mrs. G. receives 4 doses daily, how much medication will she receive per dose?
   a. 75 mg.
   b. 100 mg.
   c. 125 mg.
   d. 150 mg.

4. Which of the following medications may be administered concurrently with amphotericin B to try and minimize the adverse reactions to this medication?

   a. Analgesics.

   b. Antipyretics and antiemetics.

   c. Beta adrenergic blockers.

   d. Steroids and diuretics.

5. Mr. J. is receiving intravenous miconazole (Monistat). He should be observed for

   a. anemia.

   b. an elevated BUN.

   c. confusion.

   d. diarrhea.

6. Which of the following statements by Mr. B. leads you to believe that he has understood the teaching that you have done regarding amphotericin B (Fungizone)?

   a. "I know that as a result of taking this medication, I could develop diabetes."

   b. "I know that as a result of taking this medication, I could develop liver necrosis."

   c. "I know that as a result of taking this medication, I could develop renal damage."

   d. "I know that as a result of taking this medication, I could develop pancreatitis."

7. Which of the following medications, if administered concurrently with griseofulvin (Fulvicin), will alter its effects?

   a. Gentamicin (Garamycin).

   b. Furosemide (Lasix).

   c. Prednisone (Deltasone).

   d. Digoxin (Lanoxin).

8. Nystatin (Mycostatin) is ordered for Mrs. C. as a "swish." How should it be administered?

   a. Mrs. C. should rinse her mouth with the medication then swallow it.

   b. Mrs. C. should rinse her mouth, then spit the medication out.

   c. Mrs. C. should swallow the medication followed by 8 ounces of water.

   d. The medication should be diluted and Mrs. C. should gargle with it.

9. Which of the following would be most effective in treating tinea pedis?

   a. Acrisorcin (Akrinol).

   b. Flucytosine (Ancobon).

   c. Natamycin (Natacyn).

   d. Zinc undecylenate (Desenex).

10. The physician has ordered clotrimazole (Lotrimin) for Mrs. J.'s vaginal candidiasis. Which of the following instructions will you give Mrs. J. regarding the administration of Lotrimin?

    a. Fill the applicator with the medication and insert it into the vagina at bedtime.

    b. Apply the medication to the perineal area twice a day.

    c. Place the solution in a sitz bath and soak in it twice daily.

    d. Fill the applicator with the medication and insert into the vagina q4h and apply a sterile pad afterward.

## Critical thinking case study

M., a 32-year-old model, comes to the physician's office with fungal infection of her fingernails caused by the application of ceramic fingernails. The physician orders griseofulvin (Fulvicin). M. is leaving for a job in Hawaii and asks for a 4-week supply of the medication.

1. Discuss with M. why her plans concern you.

2.  Identify the instructions that you will give M. including the adverse effects of griseofulvin (Fulvicin).

3.  Identify three nursing diagnoses for M.

M. returns after her trip to Hawaii, complaining of headache, dizziness, and fatigue.

4.  Identify what you will do.

# CHAPTER 44

# Antiparasitics

## True or false

_____ 1. *Entamoeba histolytica* can live outside of the body for long periods.

_____ 2. Amebiasis can result in abscesses of the lungs and brain.

_____ 3. Malaria is the most common cause of mortality and morbidity worldwide.

_____ 4. Giardiasis is transmitted by the ingestion of improperly cooked beef, pork, or fish.

_____ 5. Roundworms, caused by *Ascaris lumbricoides,* are the most common parasite worm infections in the U.S.

_____ 6. Scabies and pediculosis can be transmitted by direct contact with the personal effects of an infected person.

_____ 7. Parasitic worms can enter the bloodstream and migrate to other body tissues.

_____ 8. Pyrvinium pamoate (Povan) stains feces a bright blue and can be mistaken for blood.

_____ 9. Lindane (Kwell), used for the treatment of scabies, is absorbed through the skin and can produce CNS toxicity.

_____ 10. Pyrimethamine (Daraprim) is used to treat malaria attacks.

_____ 11. Visible skin lesions associated with scabies are commonly found between the fingers.

_____ 12. Emetine hydrochloride is contraindicated for use in diabetes, liver, and respiratory disease.

_____ 13. When a trichomoniasus infection is diagnosed, it is common practice to treat the sexual partner as well as the individual with the confirmed diagnosis.

_____ 14. Quinine can also be used for treatment of nocturnal leg cramps.

_____ 15. A person being treated for dwarf tapeworms with niclosamide (Niclocide) is not considered cured until he or she has negative stools for 3 months.

## Review questions

1. During treatment of amebiasis with emetine hydrochloride, the nurse should be assessing the client for
   a. tachycardia and hypotension.
   b. oliguria and weight gain.
   c. upper gastrointestinal bleeding.
   d. convulsions and paresthesias.

2. Persons using gamma benzene hexachloride (Kwell) should be instructed to report which of the following signs/symptoms to their physician?
   a. Fatigue, cough, or dizziness.
   b. Irritation, rash, or inflammation.
   c. Headache, nausea, or diarrhea.
   d. Anorexia, nausea, or vomiting.

3. Which of the following instructions should you give to a person who is starting on gamma benzene hexachloride (Kwell)?

    a. Bathe, apply lotion to all body surfaces except head and neck, leave on for 12–24 hours, and bathe again.
    b. Apply lotion three times a day for 1 week.

    c. Take a warm shower in the morning, apply lotion all over your body, and repeat the treatment before you go to bed.
    d. Wear gloves when applying the lotion to your body and keep it away from your eyes.

4. For which of the following diagnoses should thiabendazole (Mintezol) be used with caution?

    a. Hypothyroidism.
    b. Hypertension.

    c. Renal insufficiency.
    d. Diabetes mellitus.

5. Which of the following statements by Miss B. leads you to believe that she has understood the teaching that you have done regarding metronidazole (Flagyl)?

    a. "I will refrain from operating heavy machinery while I am taking this medication."
    b. "I will avoid foods high in vitamin C."

    c. "I will not drink alcohol when I am using this medication."
    d. "I will contact my physician if I have diarrhea."

6. Which of the following foods, if taken with chloroquine phosphate (Aralen), will alter its effects?

    a. Citrus fruits.
    b. Red meats.

    c. Whole grain wheat products.
    d. Dark green leafy vegetables.

7. Mr. B. is being treated for *Pneumocystis carini* pneumonia with pentamidine isethionate (NebuPent). The following will be performed to assess the client for adverse effects of the medication:

    a. CBC.
    b. Serum potassium.

    c. Daily blood pressure.
    d. Daily weight.

8. Mr. B. is receiving quinine for malaria. He should be observed for cinchonism, symptoms of which include

    a. nausea, vomiting, and diarrhea.
    b. headache, tinnitus, and blurred vision.

    c. chest pain, dyspnea, and tachycardia.
    d. weakness, anorexia, and paresthesia.

9. Chloroquine (Aralen) should be administered

    a. on an empty stomach.
    b. with 8 ounces of water.

    c. with meals.
    d. with orange juice followed by 8 ounces of water.

10. Mrs. C., who is being treated with pyrvinium pamoate (Povan) for pinworms, called to tell you there is blood in her feces. What is the best response to Mrs. C.?

    a. "Come in immediately and we will do a stool specimen."
    b. "Don't be alarmed. We expect that your feces will change colors."

    c. "Make sure that you eat foods high in roughage and this will pass."
    d. "Povan is a dye that colors the feces bright red. Is that the color of your feces?"

## Critical thinking case study

Mrs. N., a newly married nurse on 6NW, contracts scabies from a person she has cared for on her unit. The hospital physician orders Kwell lotion.

1. Identify the instructions you will give Mrs. N. regarding the medication.

2. Identify the instruction you will give her regarding work.

Despite several treatments with Kwell, Mrs. N. still has scabies. She wonders if she should continue to use the medication.

3. Describe your response.

# SECTION VII

# Drugs Affecting the Immune System

## CHAPTER 45

## Physiology of the Immune System

### Matching exercise: terms and concepts

_____ 1. A generalized reaction to cellular injury from any cause.

_____ 2. Stimulates production of antibodies that destroy foreign invaders.

_____ 3. Detects and eliminates foreign substances that may cause tissue injury.

_____ 4. Develops during gestation or afterbirth; may be active or passive.

_____ 5. Occurs when antibodies are formed by the immune system of another person or animal and transferred to the host.

_____ 6. Foreign substances that initiate immune responses.

_____ 7. WBCs found throughout the body in lymphoma tissues.

_____ 8. The first WBCs that start phagocytosis.

_____ 9. WBCs that arrive later, ingest larger amounts of antigen, and have a longer life span.

_____ 10. The primary regulator of immune response.

_____ 11. Originate in stem cells in bone marrow.

_____ 12. Protein growth factors secreted by WBCs that stimulate leukocyte replication and function.

_____ 13. Interfere with the ability of viruses in infected cells to replicate.

_____ 14. Stimulate growth and differentiation of cells.

_____ 15. A factor that affects immunologic response.

A. Immune response.

B. Passive immunity.

C. Antigen.

D. Inflammation.

E. Immune cells.

F. T lymphocytes.

G. Interferons.

H. Immune system.

I. Cytokines.

J. Acquired immunity.

K. Interleukins.

L. Monocytes.

M. Age.

N. B lymphocytes.

O. Neutrophils.

## Review questions

1. Passive nonspecific immunity
   a. occurs when antibodies are formed by the immune system of another person and transferred to the host.
   b. develops within 6 months after birth.
   c. occurs when foreign substances stimulate production of antibodies.
   d. develops when antibodies, which are innate to the organism,being stimulated to produce WBCs.

2. The function of lymphokines is to
   a. stimulate the growth of bone marrow.
   b. suppress T cell production.
   c. inhibit protein production.
   d. stimulate production of antibodies.

3. A generalized response to cellular injury is
   a. decreased pH.
   b. increased protein catabolism.
   c. inhibition of cell growth.
   d. inflammation.

4. Cytoxic T cells act in the following ways:
   a. Secrete a toxic substance that kills the antigens.
   b. Bind to antigens and damage their cell membrane.
   c. Inject fluid into the antigen cell, causing edema and death.
   d. Decrease the activities of the B cells.

5. Which of the following immunoglobulins is located in the tissues and thought to be responsible for allergic reactions?
   a. IgG.
   b. IgA.
   c. IgM.
   d. IgE.

6. Protein growth factors, secreted by WBCs, that regulate tissue inflammation and repair and immune response are
   a. interferons.
   b. interleukins.
   c. cytokines.
   d. monocytes.

7. Interferons
   a. stimulate B lymphocyte activity.
   b. interfere with multiplication of stem cells.
   c. stimulate growth and differentiation of lymphoid cells into lymphocytes.
   d. interfere with the ability of viruses in infected cells to replicate.

8. The levels of which of the following immunoglobulins is higher at birth than at 6 months of age?
   a. IgG.
   b. IgA.
   c. IgM.
   d. IgD.

9. Which of the following has the greatest impact on the immune system?
   a. Sodium deficiency.
   b. Potassium excess.
   c. Magnesium excess.
   d. Zinc deficiency.

10. Administering immunizations
    a. strengthens antigens.
    b. suppresses the normal response to antigens.
    c. helps clients develop a tolerance to certain substances.
    d. decreases the numbers of T lymphocytes.

# CHAPTER 46

# Immunizing Agents

## Complete the following sentences

1. Immunity is the _____.

2. Active immunity develops as a result of an exposure to an _____ and results in _____. Active immunity may be _____ or _____.

3. Passive immunity occurs when _____ are formed exogenously and transferred to the host. Passive immunity lasts only _____.

4. Vaccines and toxoids are generally contraindicated in persons with _____, _____, _____, _____, _____ _____, and during _____.

5. Tetanus toxoid should be administered every _____ years in adults.

6. The following vaccines are not routinely administered to Americans unless they are traveling abroad: a. _____ b. _____ c. _____

7. Hepatitis B vaccine is recommended for those persons who are at high risk for contracting the disease, including:_____, _____, _____, _____, _____, and _____.

8. DTP (diphtheria, tetanus, and pertussis) and polio-virus vaccine should be administered at ages _____, _____, _____, _____, and _____.

9. MMR (measles, mumps, and rubella) is administered at _____.

10. _____ vaccine is recommended for older adults.

11. Before you administer a DTP you should check the person's _____.

12. If your client experiences an allergic reaction from the administration of an immunizing agent, _____ should be administered immediately.

13. Persons receiving a DTP injection may experience _____ and _____ at the injection site. They should be instructed to take _____ for symptomatic relief.

14. _____ is a rare reaction to oral polio-virus vaccine.

15. Urticaria, fever, arthralgia, and enlarged lymph nodes are symptoms of _____ which can occur _____ or _____ after an injection.

## Review questions

1. Administration of vaccines and toxoids is generally contraindicated in persons who
   a. have renal impairment.
   b. have hepatic failure.
   c. are receiving steroids.
   d. are over 65.

2. Before administering a DTP vaccine you should check the client's
   a. temperature.
   b. pulse.
   c. blood pressure.
   d. respiration.

3. You should instruct the parents of a child receiving an immunization that it is common for children to experience
   a. nausea, vomiting, and diarrhea.
   b. rash and swelling.
   c. weakness and difficulty in walking.
   d. tenderness and redness at the site.

4. Persons who have been immunized can develop serum sickness
   a. within minutes after the injection.
   b. 12 hours after the injection.
   c. days or weeks after the injection.
   d. 2–3 months after the injection.

5. MMR (measles, mumps, and rubella) is administered initially at
   a. 1–2 months of age.
   b. 3–4 months of age.
   c. 5–6 months of age.
   d. 12–15 months of age.

6. Tetanus toxoid should be administered to adults every
   a. year.
   b. 2 years.
   c. 5 years.
   d. 10 years.

7. All of the following immunizations are routinely administered to American children *except*
   a  rubella and mumps vaccine.
   b. polio-virus vaccine.
   c. diphtheria, pertussis, and tetanus.
   d. tuberculosis vaccine.

8. Hepatitis B vaccine was initially recommended for
   a. children under the age of 15.
   b. persons on dialysis or who have a renal transplant.
   c. persons with diabetes mellitus.
   d. persons over the age of 65.

9. A rare reaction resulting from the administration of polio-virus vaccine is:
   a. Myasthenia gravis.
   b. convulsions.
   c. Huntington's chorea.
   d. Guillain–Barré syndrome.

10. Anaphylaxis is most likely to occur within how many minutes after an immunizing agent is injected?
    a. 1 minute.
    b. 5 minutes.
    c. 30 minutes.
    d. 90 minutes.

## Critical thinking case study

S., a 6-month-old infant, has come to the clinic to receive her immunizations. Her mother states that S. had a reaction after her last immunization and that she does not want S. to have any more immunizations.

1. Identify the questions you should ask the mother.

2. Identify the information you should give S.'s mother regarding immunizations.

S.'s mother agrees to allow S. to have the immunization.

3. Identify what assessment should be done prior to administering the DTP vaccine and for what reasons you would withhold an immunization.

4. Instruct S.'s mom when she should return to the clinic for her daughter's next immunization.

S.'s mother calls the office to report that S. has a lump on her leg where she received the immunization.

5. Describe the advice you would give S.'s mother.

# CHAPTER 47

# Immunostimulants

## Matching exercise: terms and concepts

_____ 1. A hormone that stimulates production of RBCs.

_____ 2. Stimulates bone marrow to produce WBCs.

_____ 3. Decreased production of neutrophils.

_____ 4. Used with persons undergoing bone marrow transplantation.

_____ 5. Approved for the treatment of Kaposi's sarcoma.

_____ 6. Approved for the treatment of renal carcinoma.

_____ 7. An immunizing agent against tuberculosis, also used for bladder cancer.

_____ 8. Normal white blood cell count.

_____ 9. A mood-stabilizing agent that mobilizes neutrophils and is sometimes given to persons with chemotherapy-induced neutropenia.

_____ 10. An antiviral drug that indirectly improves immunologic function.

A. 5,000–10,000/mm$^3$.

B. Epoetin alfa (Epogen).

C. 15,000–25,000/mm$^3$.

D. Filgrastim.

E. Bacillus Calmette-Guérin (BCG).

F. Neutropenia.

G. Interleukin-2 (Aldesleukin).

H. Sargramostim.

I. Interferon-alpha 2b.

J. Lithium.

K. Levamisole (Ergamisol).

## True or false

_____ 1. Interferons can only be administered by injection.

_____ 2. Immunostimulants are used exclusively for persons with cancer.

_____ 3. Interferons should not be administered to persons who have hepatitis.

_____ 4. Toxicity from the administration of interleukin-2 (aldesleukin) can result in hard-to-control seizures.

_____ 5. Isolation procedures must be instituted if the neutrophil count drops below 500/mm$^3$.

## Crossword puzzle

**Across**

1. Any previous infections should be resolved before beginning therapy with this drug.
3. This type of drug is given only by injection.
4. Low _____ count places the patient at risk of infection.
6. Interferon-alfa-n3 is approved only for treatment of recurring _____.
8. Stimulates granulocyte production.
9. An abnormal decrease in white blood cells.

**Down**

2. Given after bone marow transplantation via slow IV.
5. An abbreviation for the immunostimulant that can cause bladder cancer remission.
7. This type of tumor in the breast, lung, or colon does not respond to interferon.

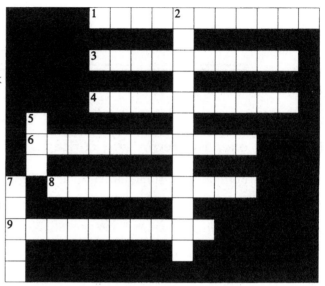

## Review questions

1. Mr. G. is undergoing a bone marrow transplant. The drug that will be most effective in stimulating the production of granulocytes and macrophages is
   a. Bacillus Calmette-Guérin (BCG).
   b. epoetin alfa (Epogen).
   c. filgrastin.
   d. sargramostim.

2. Which of the following is considered a toxic side effect of interleukin-2 (aldesleukin) and would necessitate discontinuation of the drug?
   a. BP of 150/90.
   b. Repetitive seizures.
   c. Blood sugar 300 mg/dl
   d. Confusion.

3. Mr. G. has just had a bone marrow transplant. Which of the following nursing diagnoses would take priority?
   a. Body image disturbance related to illness.
   b. High risk for infection related to immunosuppression.
   c. Anxiety related to diagnosis of cancer.
   d. Activity intolerance related to fatigue.

4. Immunostimulants are being administered to Mr. C. to increase his WBC to
   a. 2000–5000/mm$^3$.
   b. 5000–10,000/mm$^3$.
   c. 1500–2000/mm$^3$.
   d. 2000–2400/mm$^3$.

5. An expected outcome after the administration of epoetin alfa (Epogen) is
   a. decreased RBC count.
   b. increased RBC count.
   c. increased WBC count.
   d. decreased WBC count.

6. One of the adverse effects of the anti-AIDS drug zidovudine (Retrovir) that the nurse needs to assess for is
   a. decreased WBC count.
   b. increased WBC count.
   c. decreased RBC count.
   d. increased RBC count.

7. Which of the following statements by Mr. G., who has renal carcinoma, leads you to believe that he has understood the teaching that you have done regarding interleukin-2 (aldesleukin)?

   a. "This drug will inhibit tumor growth."
   b. "This drug will prevent me from developing a viral infection."
   c. "This drug will decrease the number of T cells."
   d. "This drug can cause renal failure."

8. For which of the following individuals would the use of BCG for bladder cancer be contraindicated?

   a. A person with a history of heart disease.
   b. A person with a history of diabetes mellitus.
   c. A person with a history of pulmonary fibrosis.
   d. A person with a history of a renal transplant.

9. For persons who are immunosuppressed, the following lifestyle change will enhance their immune mechanisms:

   a. Eliminate fats and sugar from diet.
   b. Increase vitamin C in diet.
   c. Avoid usage of tobacco and alcohol.
   d. Exercise daily.

10. An expected outcome after the administration of immunostimulants is

    a. an RBC of 3000/mm$^3$.
    b. decreased numbers or severity of infections.
    c. increased life expectancy.
    d. a WBC of 20,000/mm$^3$.

## Critical thinking case study

Mr. J., a 36-year-old accountant, is to receive a bone marrow transplant. He will be receiving sargramostim after the procedure to promote bone marrow function.

1. Discuss the teaching that you will do with Mr. J. and his wife.

2. Identify the assessments that you will do.

Mr. J. is very nervous after the transplant and asks you if the graft has been successful.

3. Identify how you will respond to Mr. J.'s inquiry.

# CHAPTER 48

# Immunosuppressants

## True or false

_____ 1. Rheumatoid arthritis results from an inappropriate activation of the immune response.

_____ 2. Acute organ rejection occurs within 2 days following transplantation.

_____ 3. Once an individual has had a transplanted organ for a year, he or she will not experience organ rejection.

_____ 4. Corticosteroids increase the numbers of circulating basophils, eosinophils, and monocytes.

_____ 5. Cytotoxic antimetabolites block cellular reproduction.

_____ 6. Methotrexate (Rheumatrex) has been used to treat severe psoriasis.

_____ 7. Cyclosporine (Sandimmune) is used to prevent graft-versus-host disease in transplant recipients.

_____ 8. Antithymocyte globulin (ATG) should not be administered to persons who have an allergy to cow serum.

_____ 9. Isolation techniques are instituted for transplant recipients whose neutrophil count drops below 1000/mm³.

_____ 10. Immediately following a transplant, the recipient is allowed no visitors in order to prevent infection.

_____ 11. Persons taking immunosuppressants should avoid the use of alcohol and tobacco.

_____ 12. Lymphoma may result from immunosuppression.

_____ 13. Persons receiving methotrexate (Rheumatrex) should have liver function studies performed monthly.

_____ 14. The preferred route for administering cyclosporine (Sandimmune) is parenterally because it is more effective.

_____ 15. Symptoms of neurotoxicity produced by cyclosporine include confusion, hallucinations, and seizures.

## Review questions

1. One adverse effect of excessive immunosuppression is the development of
   a. liver failure.
   b. kidney failure.
   c. Kaposi's sarcoma.
   d. serious infection.

2. Which of the following statements by 8-year-old BJ leads you to believe that she has a good understanding of how to take cyclosporine (Sandimmune)?
   a. "I will take cyclosporine (Sandimmune) on an empty stomach."
   b. "I will follow the cyclosporine (Sandimmune) with 8 ounces of water."
   c. "I will rinse out the glass after I have taken the cyclosporine (Sandimmune) and drink the rinse solution."
   d. "I will only take the medication after meals."

3. Persons receiving azathioprine (Imuran) should be observed for

   a. respiratory distress.
   b. depression.

   c. abnormal bleeding.
   d. severe diarrhea.

4. Mr. J., who is receiving antithymocyte globulin (ATG) (Atgam), experiences chest pain and difficulty in breathing. Your initial nursing action should be to

   a. stop the drug infusion.
   b. slow down the drug infusion.

   c. contact the physician.
   d. administer oxygen and nitroglycerin.

5. Which of the following medications, if administered concurrently with cyclosporine (Sandimmune), will decrease its effect?

   a. Verapamil (Calan).
   b. Phenytoin (Dilantin).

   c. Cimetidine (Tagamet).
   d. Gentamicin (Garamycin)

6. Which of the following instructions should be given to Mr. H. who is receiving methotrexate (Rheumatrex) to help him avoid the adverse effects of the medication?

   a. Increase the fiber in your diet.
   b. Walk at least a mile every day and get a good night's sleep.

   c. Drink at least 8 glasses of water daily.
   d. Wear protective clothing and use sunscreen to decrease your exposure to the sun.

7. A nursing diagnosis that the nurse needs to include in Mrs. J.'s care plan after a renal transplant has been performed is:

   a. Social isolation.
   b. Impaired gas exchange.

   c. Impaired cardiac output.
   d. Activity intolerance.

8. Mr. P. is receiving immunosuppressive agents after a heart transplant. For which one of the following assessments would you contact the physician?

   a. Weight loss of 3 lbs.
   b. Temperature of 36.8°C.

   c. Productive cough.
   d. Hypoactive bowel sounds.

9. After his liver transplant, Mr. J. receives immunosuppressants to prevent the following complication:

   a. Ascites.
   b. Septicemia.

   c. Organ rejection.
   d. Clotting off of graft.

10. Persons receiving immunosuppressants after a kidney transplant should be observed for deterioration in kidney function. Which of the following lab studies would give you the earliest indication of a change in renal status?

    a. BUN.
    b. Serum sodium.

    c. Serum potassium.
    d. Creatinine clearance.

## Critical thinking case study

M.B., a 12-year-old who received a kidney transplant yesterday, is taking cyclosporine (Sandimmune) and prednisone (Deltasone) to prevent rejection of the transplanted organ. (The learner may need to use additional sources to answer this question.)

1. Identify what you will be assessing for and your rationale for each assessment.

2.  Identify the teaching that you will do regarding the medications M.B. is taking.

M.B.'s urinary output is minimal and her physician decides to dialyze her. M.B. starts crying, stating, "I've lost my kidney, haven't I?"

3.  Describe the best response to M.B.'s statement.

# SECTION VIII

# Drugs Affecting the Respiratory System

---

## CHAPTER 49

## Physiology of the Respiratory System

---

## Matching exercise: terms and concepts

_____ 1. Permanent damage results when tissues are deprived of oxygen for this length of time.

_____ 2. Hairlike projections that sweep mucus toward the pharynx.

_____ 3. The right lung contains this.

_____ 4. The functional units of the lungs.

_____ 5. This lining adheres to the surface of the lung.

_____ 6. The outer layer of the lung that lines the thoracic cavity.

_____ 7. The ability of the lungs to stretch or expand.

_____ 8. Regulates the rate and depth of respiration.

_____ 9. This stimulates the respiratory center.

_____ 10. The normal percentage of oxygen contained in room air.

_____ 11. Average tidal volume.

_____ 12. A sigh occurs.

_____ 13. Causes bronchodilation.

_____ 14. Gas exchange occurs here.

_____ 15. Responsible for carrying $O_2$.

A. Oxygen level.

B. Carbon dioxide.

C. Visceral pleura.

D. 4–6 minutes.

E. 2–3 minutes.

F. Cilia.

G. Three lobes.

H. Two lobes.

I. Lobules.

J. Parietal pleura.

K. Compliance.

L. Medulla oblongata.

M. Pons.

N. 21%.

O. Cerebellum.

P. 35%.

Q. 1–2 times per hour.

R. 6–10 times per hour.

S. 500 ml.

T. 700 ml.

U. Parasympathetic nervous system.

V. Sympathetic nervous system.

W. Trachea.

X. Alveoli.

Y. White blood cells.

Z. Hemoglobin.

## Review questions

1. Which of the following causes an increased respiratory rate?

   a. Increased $pCO_2$.

   b. Decreased $pCO_2$.

   c. Increased $O_2$.

   d. Decreased pH.

2. Which of the following disease processes would have the most significant impact on decreasing the compliance of the lungs?

   a. Pulmonary fibrosis.

   b. Pneumonia.

   c. Anemia.

   d. Cerebellar injury.

3. The percentage of oxygen in room air is

   a. 21%.

   b. 28%.

   c. 35%.

   d. 40%.

4. Air exchange takes place in

   a. the trachea.

   b. the bronchioles.

   c. the alveoli.

   d. all of the above.

5. Which of the following disease processes would have an impact on perfusion?

   a. Hypertension.

   b. Anemia.

   c. Cerebral vascular accident.

   d. Pneumonia.

6. You would document the breathing pattern of a person with a respiratory rate of 12 as

   a. normopnea.

   b. tachypnea.

   c. bradypnea.

   d. apnea.

7. Mr. J. takes in 500 ml of air with each breath. This is referred to as

   a. total lung capacity.

   b. residual volume.

   c. vital capacity.

   d. tidal volume.

8. Which of the following regulates the rate and depth of respiration?

   a. Cerebrum.

   b. Cerebellum.

   c. Medulla oblongata.

   d. Reticular activating system.

9. Which of the following is responsible for bronchodilation?

   a. Parasympathetic nervous system.

   b. Sympathetic nervous system.

   c. Medulla oblongata.

   d. Cerebrum.

10. Permanent damage can occur when the brain is deprived of oxygen for

    a. 1 minute.

    b. 2 minutes.

    c. 3 minutes.

    d. 4 minutes.

# CHAPTER 50

# Bronchodilating and Antiasthmatic Drugs

## Matching exercise: terms and concepts

____  1. Bronchodilators that also have a mild diuretic effect.

____  2. Reduces intracellular GMP, a bronchoconstricting substance.

____  3. Reduces inflammation and mucus secretion.

____  4. Stimulate receptors in bronchial smooth muscle to produce bronchodilation.

A.  Adrenergic.

B.  Xanthines.

C.  Anticholinergics.

D.  Corticosteroids.

## Complete the following sentences

1. Bronchoconstriction may be precipitated by:

   a. _____.
   b. _____.
   c. _____.
   d. _____.
   e. _____.
   f. _____.
   g. _____.
   h. _____.
   i. _____.

2. Epinephrine (_____) is administered for an _____.
   The therapeutic effects will be seen in _____.

3. Albuterol (_____) can be administered _____ or by _____.

4. Ipratropium bromide (_____) improves pulmonary function within ___ minutes. The common adverse effects seen with this drug are _____, _____, _____, _____, _____, and _____.

5. Beclomethasone (_____) (_____) and triamcinolone (_____) are corticosteroids and are administered by _____.

6. Theophylline comes in _____ acting and _____ acting preparations.

7. Cromolyn (____) is effective in treating _____ and _____.

8. Severe respiratory distress is characterized by _____, _____, _____, and _____.

9. Early signs of hypoxia include: _____, _____, _____,

     _____, and _____.

10. Clients with chronic obstructive pulmonary disease should drink _____ ml/day to

     _____. They should also avoid excessive caffeine because this may increase

     _____ and _____.

11. When using an inhaler you should

     a. _____.
     b. _____.
     c. _____.
     d. _____.

     e. _____.
     f. _____.
     g. _____.
     h. _____.

12. If you are administering two inhalers, a bronchodilator and a corticosteroid, which one should you

     give first? _____.

13. After inhalation of a corticosteroid, the client should rinse his or her mouth. This will help prevent

     a _____.

## True or false

_____ 1. Children require a lower dose of theophylline.

_____ 2. Cigarette smokers require a higher dose of theophylline.

_____ 3. The physician needs to know the body weight of the client before he or she can determine
         the correct dosage of theophylline.

_____ 4. Theophylline can cause bradycardia.

_____ 5. If an individual has congestive heart failure he or she may require a higher dose of theophylline.

_____ 6. If an individual is already taking cimetidine (Tagamet) and is started on theophylline, the
         dosage of theophylline will need to be decreased.

## Review questions

1. M. is newly diagnosed with asthma. She should be instructed to avoid which of the following
   because they may cause her to experience bronchoconstriction?
   a. Becoming fatigued.
   b. Direct sunlight.
   c. Extremely cold temperatures.
   d. Foods high in sodium.

2. Mr. H. may need to have his dosage of theophylline increased if he
   a. uses insulin.
   b. takes cimetidine (Tagamet).
   c. exercises strenuously.
   d. smokes cigarettes.

3. Mr. B. is started on oral theophylline. You know that your teaching has been successful if he states
   the following:
   a. "I will limit my intake of caffeine."
   b. "I know that I should eat foods high in
      potassium."
   c. "I will not drink more than 1000 ml of
      water a day."
   d. "I will take the medicine on an
      empty stomach."

4. Mrs. B. is started on an albuterol (Proventil) inhaler. You should observe her for

    a. polydipsia.
    b. tachycardia.
    c. hypotension.
    d. diarrhea.

5. Which of the following statements indicates that Mr. G. has a good understanding of the teaching that you have done regarding inhalers?

    a. "I should inhale before administering a puff."
    b. "The aerosol canister should be shaken well before using."
    c. "I need to take three short quick breaths when I administer the inhaler."
    d. "I cannot administer a second aerosol medication until 30 minutes after the first aerosol medication."

6. Which of the following drugs is effective in treating acute bronchospasm?

    a. Ipratropium bromide (Atrovent).
    b. Epinephrine (Adrenalin).
    c. Cromolyn (Intal).
    d. Ephedrine.

7. A client with chronic bronchitis is experiencing symptoms of respiratory distress. Which of the following symptoms indicate hypoxia?

    a. Excessive mucus production.
    b. Expiratory wheezes and cyanosis.
    c. Activity intolerance.
    d. Increased pulse and blood pressure.

8. To avoid bronchospasm, the person who experiences acute asthma attacks should be advised to

    a. use inhalers prior to exercise.
    b. avoid all strenuous exercise.
    c. avoid all stressful situations.
    d. limit time outdoors to 1 hour per day.

9. All of the following are helpful in removing secretions from the respiratory tract *except*

    a. drinking 2000 ml daily.
    b. postural drainage.
    c. deep breathing.
    d. administration of corticosteroids.

10. A drug that increases the effectiveness of bronchodilators is

    a. lithium (Eskalith).
    b. phenobarbital (Luminal).
    c. propranolol (Inderal).
    d. cimetidine (Tagamet).

# CHAPTER 51

# Antihistamines

## Matching exercise: terms and concepts

_____ 1. Used as an antipruritic in allergic and nonallergic pruritus.

_____ 2. Used to prevent motion sickness.

_____ 3. May affect blood pressure when given parenterally.

_____ 4. Given parenterally for treatment of allergic reactions to blood.

_____ 5. A very potent antihistamine that produces significant sedation.

_____ 6. Weight gain has been reported in persons taking this drug.

_____ 7. Should not be used in persons with asthma.

_____ 8. Has antihistamine, antiemetic, antianxiety, and sedative effects.

_____ 9. A combination product containing an antihistamine, an adrenergic agent, and other ingredients.

_____ 10. An adverse effect of the administration of antihistamines.

_____ 11. A newer antihistamine that does not produce drowsiness.

_____ 12. When antihistamines are administered for their antiemetic effect, you should see a decrease in this symptom.

A. Promethazine hydrochloride (Phenergan).

B. Methdilazine (Tacaryl).

C. Dimenhydrinate (Dramamine).

D. Drowsiness.

E. Diphenhydramine hydrochloride (Benadryl).

F. Cyproheptadine (Periactin).

G. Chlorpheniramine maleate (Chlor-Trimeton).

H. Azatadine maleate (Optimine).

I. Dimetapp.

J. Hydroxyzine (Vistaril).

K. Headache.

L. Terfenadine (Seldane).

M. Dizziness.

N. Nausea and vomiting.

## Review questions

1. Which of the following statements by Mrs. H. indicates successful teaching concerning diphenhydramine hydrochloride (Benadryl)?
   a. "I can still have my after-dinner drink."
   b. "I will eat a diet high in roughage while I am taking this medication."
   c. "I should not operate heavy machinery when I take this medicine."
   d. "I can take this medication as frequently as I need it."

2. Antihistamines should be used with caution in individuals who have
   a. Parkinson's disease.
   b. hypertension.
   c. diabetes mellitus.
   d. prostatic hypertrophy.

3. Which of the following conditions in Mrs. G.'s history could contraindicate the use of phenothiazines?
   a. Colostomy.
   b. Mitral valve prolapse.
   c. Depression.
   d. Thyroid disease.

4. Persons taking brompheniramine maleate (Dimetane) should be given the following instructions:

    a. Do not drink more than 1500 ml daily.
    b. Only take the medication at bedtime.
    c. Eat foods high in vitamin C while you are taking this medication.
    d. Avoid the use of alcohol while you are using this medication.

5. The physician ordered meclizine hydrochloride (Antivert) for Mrs. B. with Ménière's disease. Common adverse effects of this medication include

    a. dizziness and headache.
    b. urinary retention and constipation.
    c. dry mouth and blurred vision.
    d. diarrhea and abdominal cramping.

6. When diphenhydramine hydrochloride (Benadryl) is administered parenterally, the nurse needs to observe the client for changes in

    a. heart rate.
    b. blood pressure.
    c. respiratory rate.
    d. orientation.

7. Which of the following antihistamines is also effective as an antiemetic?

    a. Astemizole (Hismanal).
    b. Clemastine fumarate (Tavist).
    c. Hydroxyzine hydrochloride (Atarax).
    d. Trimeprazine tartrate (Temaril).

8. An expected outcome after the administration of cyproheptadine (Periactin) is

    a. weight gain.
    b. increased urinary output.
    c. decreased anxiety.
    d. decreased blood pressure.

9. An overdose of antihistamines can result in

    a. a myocardial infarction.
    b. a hypertensive crisis.
    c. liver failure.
    d. hallucinations and convulsions.

10. The physician has ordered diphenhydramine hydrocholoride (Benadryl) for sleep for Mr. G., an 80-year-old man who lives with his daughter. Which of the following adverse effects should Mr. G.'s daughter be watching for?

    a. Constipation.
    b. Urinary retention.
    c. Tachycardia.
    d. Drowsiness.

## Critical thinking case study

Mrs. J. is a 55-year-old woman recently diagnosed with Ménière's disease. The physician orders meclizine hydrochloride (Antivert). (The learner may need additional sources to answer the questions below.)

1. Discuss with Mrs. J. the reason the medication was ordered and the potential adverse effects.

Mrs. J. is very distressed about her diagnosis and asks you if there are any other medications that will help her.

2. Identify your response.

Mrs. J. asks you what restrictions she will have.

3. Identify how you will respond to her.

# CHAPTER 52

# Nasal Decongestants, Antitussives, Mucolytics, and Cold Remedies

## Complete the following sentences

1. These medications are contraindicated for individuals with narrow-angle glaucoma:
   _____.

2. Coryza is _____.

3. A prominent symptom of respiratory tract infection is a _____.

4. Nonrespiratory conditions that predispose individuals to secretion retention include
   _____, _____, and _____.

5. Antitussives are used when a nonproductive cough interferes with
   _____.

6. This mucolytic is also used for treatment of acetaminophen overdosage:
   _____.

7. Ingredients used in narcotic antitussives include _____, _____,
   _____, and _____.

8. If nasal decongestants are overused, they can cause _____.

9. Nasal decongestants can _____ the heart rate and blood pressure.

10. Adverse effects associated with the use of narcotic antitussives include: _____,
    _____, _____, _____, _____,
    _____, and _____.

11. These medications should not be administered with dextromethorphan:
    _____.

12. Before instilling nasal decongestants you should have the patient
    _____.

13. Nasal decongestants should be administered to infants _____.

14. After administering cough syrups, the patient should avoid eating or drinking for
    _____.

15. Individuals who require expectorants for congestion should be encouraged to drink
    _____ daily.

## Crossword puzzle

### Across

1. A nasal decongestant.
5. A non-narcotic antitussive.
9. Many over-the-counter decongestants can decrease _____
   discharge.

### Down

2. A mucolytic.
3. An ingredient found in Dristan.
4. Inflammation of the mucous
   membrane of the nose.
5. A cold, cough, and allergy remedy.
6. An expectorant.
7. A commonly used medication for colds
   and coughs that contains guaifenesin.
8. An agent that suppresses cough by
   depressing the respiratory center.

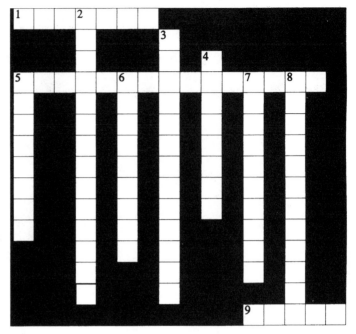

## Review questions

1. Which statement by Mr. C. would lead you to believe that he needs additional instruction regarding his nasal decongestant?

   a. "I will blow my nose before instilling the
      nasal spray."
   b. "I will report any dizziness, drowsiness ,
      or rapid pulse."
   c. "I will drink 2000–3000 ml of fluid daily."
   d. "I will use it only when I have nasal
      discharge."

2. An adverse reaction commonly experienced by persons taking nasal decongestants is

   a. diarrhea.
   b. dry mouth.
   c. rash.
   d. headache.

3. Which of the following statements by Mr. H. leads you to believe that he has understood the teaching that you have done regarding his antitussive?

   a. "I can take this medication as often
      as I need it."
   b. "It is best to take the cough syrup
      with meals."
   c. "I should be careful driving while I am
      taking this medication."
   d. "I can still have my evening cocktail as
      long as I limit it to 2 drinks."

4. Which of the following groups of medications, if administered with dextromethorphan, could cause
   apnea?

   a. Calcium channel blockers.
   b. MAO inhibitors.
   c. Beta blockers.
   d. Thiazide diuretics.

5. Which of the following medications, if administered with nasal decongestants, would increase the
   risk of cardiac arrhythmias?

   a. Atropine.
   b. Propranolol (Inderal).
   c. Theophylline (Aminophylline).
   d. Furosemide (Lasix).

6. The following instructions should be given to the mother of S.Q., a 3-month-old infant who has an upper respiratory tract infection and has been placed on nasal decongestants:

   a. Instill the medication 20-30 minutes before feeding.
   b. Keep the baby on clear liquids until the nasal discharge has resolved.
   c. Start the baby on cereal because she is having difficulty sucking right now.
   d. Give S.Q. the medication immediately before feeding, followed by 4 ounces of water.

7. Persons taking codeine phosphate, a narcotic antitussive, need to be observed for

   a. respiratory depression.
   b. constipation.
   c. tachycardia.
   d. muscle rigidity.

8. Mr. G., who has cancer of the lung, complains of a persistent cough that interrupts his sleep. Which of the following assessments should the nurse perform relative to Mr. G.'s complaint before contacting the physician to ask for an order for an antitussive?

   a. Count the number and length of each coughing spell.
   b. Count his respiratory and pulse rates for a full minute.
   c. Determine $pO_2$ levels.
   d. Observe for any sputum and evaluate its color and consistency.

9. Mr. J., who is diagnosed with pneumonia, is using acetylcysteine (Mucomyst). A nursing action that would be appropriate for Mr. J. is:

   a. discouraging Mr. J. from resting during the day.
   b. checking breath sounds every hour.
   c. maintaining Mr. J. on bed rest to avoid complications caused by Mucomyst.
   d. encourage 2000–3000 ml fluid intake daily.

10. Instructions that the nurse should give to Mr. H., who is taking saturated solution of potassium iodide (SSKI), include the following:

    a. Always take this medication on an empty stomach.
    b. Dilute the medication in a full glass of juice.
    c. Do not drink anything for an hour after this medication.
    d. This medication should be taken 20-30 minutes before meals.

## Critical thinking case study

Mr. Z., who has a 10-year history of chronic obstructive pulmonary disease, has a temperature of 103°F, congestion is audible upon auscultation, and his lung sounds are diminished in the bases bilaterally. The physician orders IV antibiotics, saturated solution of potassium iodide (SSKI), and acetylcysteine (Mucomyst). (The learner may need to use additional sources to answer these questions.)

1. Identify the instructions that you will give Mr. Z. before administering the medications.

2. Describe your nursing interventions for Mr. Z.

Mr. Z. has begun coughing up small amounts of tenacious sputum.

3. Identify your nursing actions.

4. Identify the instructions you will give Mr. Z. that may help prevent a recurrence of pneumonia

# SECTION IX

# Drugs Affecting the Cardiovascular System

---

## CHAPTER 53

## Physiology of the Cardiovascular System

---

## Matching exercise: terms and concepts

_____ 1. Receives deoxygenated blood by way of the vena cava.

_____ 2. Pumps oxygenated blood through the systemic circuit.

_____ 3. Muscle that separates the right and left sides of the heart.

_____ 4. Membrane lining the heart chambers.

_____ 5. Valve separating the right atrium and ventricle.

_____ 6. The pacemaker of the heart.

_____ 7. Responsible for increasing the heart rate.

_____ 8. The smooth inner lining of an artery.

_____ 9. Where the exchange of gases, nutrients, and waste products takes place.

_____ 10. Helps maintain colloid osmotic pressure.

_____ 11. Transports oxygen.

_____ 12. Essential to blood coagulation.

_____ 13. Functions as a defense mechanism against micro-organisms.

_____ 14. The resting or filling phase of the cardiac cycle.

_____ 15. Carry lymphocytes and large molecules of protein and fat.

A. SA node.

B. Right atrium.

C. Tricuspid valve.

D. Myocardium.

E. Left ventricle.

F. Endocardium.

G. Septum.

H. Parasympathetic nerves.

I. AV node.

J. Mitral valve.

K. Sympathetic nerves.

L. Intima.

M. Media.

N. Veins.

O. Capillaries.

P. Albumin.

Q. Hemoglobin.

R. Erythrocytes.

S. Diastolic.

T. Platelets.

U. Systolic.

V. Lymphatic vessels.

## Review questions

1. The valve that separates the left atrium and ventricle is the
   a. mitral.
   b. pulmonic.
   c. aortic.
   d. tricuspid.

2. The ability of the heart to pump efficiently depends on the client's
   a. age.
   b. venous capacitance.
   c. heart rate.
   d. blood pressure.

3. Which of the following areas of the heart can beat independently with a rate of 30–40 beats per minute?
   a. The AV node.
   b. The bundle of His.
   c. Purkinje fibers.
   d. The ventricles.

4. Red blood cells are produced by the
   a. reticulo-endothelial tissues.
   b. lymphatic tissue.
   c. bone marrow.
   d. liver.

5. The blood does all of the following *except*
   a. help regulate body temperature.
   b. transport oxygen.
   c. protect the body from invading organisms.
   d. regulate metabolism of glucose.

6. The middle layer of an artery is composed of
   a. elastic tissue.
   b. connective tissue.
   c. fibrous tissue.
   d. reticular tissue.

7. Red blood cells are also referred to as
   a. leukocytes.
   b. erythrocytes.
   c. thrombocytes.
   d. megakaryocytes.

8. The fibrous sac enclosing the heart is the
   a. endocardium.
   b. myocardium.
   c. epicardium.
   d. pericardium.

9. Vessels that carry large molecules of protein and fat are the
   a. arteries.
   b. veins.
   c. capillaries.
   d. lymphatic vessels.

10. The component of the blood necessary for maintaining colloid osmotic pressure is
    a. albumin.
    b. fibrinogen.
    c. gamma globulin.
    d. platelets.

# CHAPTER 54

# Cardiotonic-Inotropic Agents Used in Congestive Heart Failure

1. When cardiac output falls, the body attempts to compensate by increasing sympathetic activity, which _____ the force of the contraction, _____ the heart rate, and causes _____. Aldosterone is released and causes increased reabsorption of sodium and water, which _____ blood volume and _____ blood pressure, which results in _____.

2. As a result of these compensatory mechanisms there is increased _____ and increased afterload.

3. Digitalis glycosides _____ myocardial contractility and _____ the rate of ventricular contraction.

4. Digitalis is used to treat the following atrial tachyarrhythmias such as atrial _____, atrial _____, and paroxysmal atrial tachycardia or supraventricular tachycardia.

5. An oral digitalizing dose in an adult is _____ in 24 hours.

6. A child age 2, weighing 22 lbs., requires digitalization. The physician orders 0.04 mg/kg in 4 equal doses. How much medication will the child receive per dose? _____.

7. Kelly, a newborn, who weighs 5 lbs. and has tetralogy of Fallot, is started on 0.025 mg/kg of digoxin. How much medication will the child receive per day? _____.

8. Amrinone (_____) is used for _____ management of CHF not controlled by digitalis and diuretic therapy.

9. When persons are taking digoxin, hypokalemia may precipitate _____.

10. Intravenous dosage of digoxin should be _____ less than the oral dose.

11. Hypokalemia (<3.5 mEq/liter) and hypomagnesemia (<1.5–2.5 mg/100 ml) lead to _____.

12. Hypercalcemia (>8.5–10 mg/100 ml) enhances _____.

13. Hypokalemia, hypomagnesemia and hypercalcemia increase the risk of _____.

14. Adverse effects of digitalis include
    a. _____.
    b. _____.
    c. _____.
    d. _____.

15. Adverse effects from amrinone (Inocor) include

    a. _____.

    b. _____.

    c. _____.

    d. _____

## Matching exercise: Cardiovascular

____ 1. A heart rate below 60.

____ 2. A complication of acute heart failure characterized by buildup of secretions in the lungs and respiratory difficulty.

____ 3. The usual daily maintenance dose of digoxin.

____ 4. Administration of relatively large doses of digoxin.

____ 5. A drug used to treat digitalis-induced bradycardia.

____ 6. An electrolyte deviation that can increase the risk of digoxin toxicity.

____ 7. An arrhythmia in which the atrial heart rate is faster than the ventricular rate.

____ 8. An antidote for digitalis toxicity.

____ 9. A K-losing diuretic often used in the treatment of congestive heart failure.

____ 10. The route of digoxin administration used least often because it causes tissue irritation.

____ 11. A therapeutic digoxin level.

a. Digitalization.

b. Oral.

c. Premature ventricular contractions (PVCs).

d. Digoxin immune fab (Digibind).

e. Atropine.

f. Bradycardia.

g. Hypercalcemia.

h. Pulmonary edma.

i. Intramuscular.

j. Furosemide (Lasix).

k. 0.125–0.25 mg.

l. 0.5–2.0 mg/ml.

m. Atrial fibrillation.

n. Tachycardia.

## Review Questions

1. Congestive heart failure results in an increased preload which is an increased
   a. amount of venous blood returning to the heart.
   b. resistance that the heart must overcome to pump effectively.
   c. amount of blood pooled in the extremities.
   d. pulse rate caused by venous distention.

2. Mrs. G., who is taking digoxin (Lanoxin) and furosemide (Lasix), complains of a headache and nausea. Which of the following would you do first?
   a. Contact her physician immediately.
   b. Check her vital signs.
   c. Administer an antiemetic.
   d. Administer Tylenol and Maalox.

3. Mr. J. is admitted to the hospital for atrial fibrillation and is given 2 digoxin doses totaling 1 mg. You check his lab studies the next day and find his digoxin level to be 0.4 mg/ml. You know that this is
   a. lower than a therapeutic range.
   b. within a therapeutic range.
   c. higher than a therapeutic range.

4. Mrs. H. is to be discharged on 0.125 mg of digoxin daily. Which of the following statements by Mrs. H. leads you to believe she has understood your teaching?
   a. "I will take the medicine in the morning before I get out of bed."
   b. "I will take my pulse every day."
   c. "I will stop the medicine if my pulse is below 60."
   d. "I will eat a diet high in bran fiber."

5. When administering amrinone (Inocor), you should observe for the following adverse effect.

   a. Hypoglycemia.

   b. Confusion.

   c. Hypotension.

   d. Seizures.

6. Cardiac glycosides are used to

   a. decrease cardiac output.

   b. decrease afterload.

   c. increase the ventricular rate.

   d. increase the force of cardiac contraction.

7. Which of the following is an outcome associated with the administration of digoxin?

   a. Increased heart size.

   b. Increased urinary output.

   c. Decreased respiratory rate.

   d. Decreased blood sugar.

8. Persons taking digoxin (Lanoxin) and phenytoin (Dilantin) concurrently may have

   a. decreased Dilantin levels.

   b. elevated digoxin levels.

   c. decreased digoxin levels.

   d. elevated Dilantin levels.

9. When given with digoxin (Lanoxin), which of the following medications will increase the serum digoxin concentration?

   a. Nitroglycerin (NitroBid).

   b. Furosemide (Lasix).

   c. Glyburide (Diabeta).

   d. Verapamil (Calan).

10. Mr. A. is admitted with acute CHF and is to be started on digoxin (Lanoxin). Which of the following assessments is necessary before administering the initial dose?

    a. Assess Mr. A.'s respiratory status.

    b. Assess Mr. A.'s liver function.

    c. Assess Mr. A.'s kidney function.

    d. Assess Mr. A.'s blood sugar.

## Critical thinking case study

M., a 6-year-old weighing 42 lbs., is admitted to your unit for treatment of CHF. She is to be started on digoxin (Lanoxin), furosemide (Lasix), and potassium. The physician orders daily CBCs, digoxin levels, weighs and q4h vital signs.

1. Describe the digitalizing regimen to M.'s mother and what she can expect.

2. Identify the adverse effects that you plan to discuss with M.'s mother and why this information is important for her to know.

3. Describe the potential drug interactions that you will discuss with M.'s mother.

M.'s mother asks why so many tests are being performed.

4. Explain the reason for the tests in terms both mother and child can understand.

5. Identify ways of assessing compliance.

6. Identify and prioritize 3 nursing diagnoses for a child with congestive heart failure.

# CHAPTER 55

# Antiarrhythmic Drugs

## Matching exercise: terms and concepts

_____ 1. Irregular heart rate or rhythm.

_____ 2. Normal cardiac cycle.

_____ 3. Time during the cardiac cycle when the heart is unable to respond to a new stimulus.

_____ 4. The normal pacemaker of the heart.

_____ 5. An abnormal pacemaker.

_____ 6. A life-threatening arrhythmia.

_____ 7. May indicate impending heart block or cardio-vascular collapse.

_____ 8. A sign of increased cardiac output.

_____ 9. A prolonged PR interval.

_____ 10. Symptoms of induced congestive heart failure.

A. Sinus rhythm.

B. Arrhythmia or dysrhythmia.

C. Fatigue and weight gain.

D. First–degree heart block.

E. Increased urinary output.

F. Refractory period.

G. SA node.

H. AV node.

I. Second–degree heart block.

J. Ectopic focus.

K. Tachycardia.

L. Bradycardia.

M. Ventricular fibrillation.

## Crossword puzzle

**Across**

9. Initial drug of choice for atrial fibrillation.
10. Urinary retention can occur with administration of this drug.

**Down**

1. This medication should be administered with food to prevent GI upset.
2. Used to slow the ventricular rate; contraindicated in CHF.
3. A drug that increases the heart rate in bradycardia or heart block.
4. Rapid-acting drug given intra-venously for supraventricular tachycardia.
5. For short-term treatment of ventricular arrhythmias.
6. This drug is used to treat PVCs when lidocaine is ineffective.
7. Used to treat bradycardia.
8. Used to treat supraventricular tachycardia, atrial fibrillation, and atrial flutter.

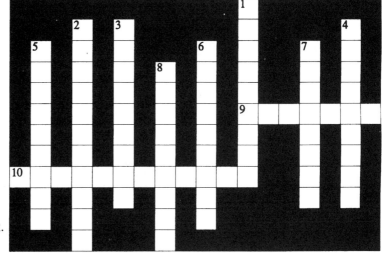

# Cardiac electrophysiology

### PART A. DIAGRAM COMPLETION

Choose a term from the following list to correctly identify the heart's conduction system as illustrated in Figure 55-1.

Left ventricle                     SA node
Purkinje fibers                    AV node
Right ventricle                    Right bundle branch
Right atrium                       Bundle of His

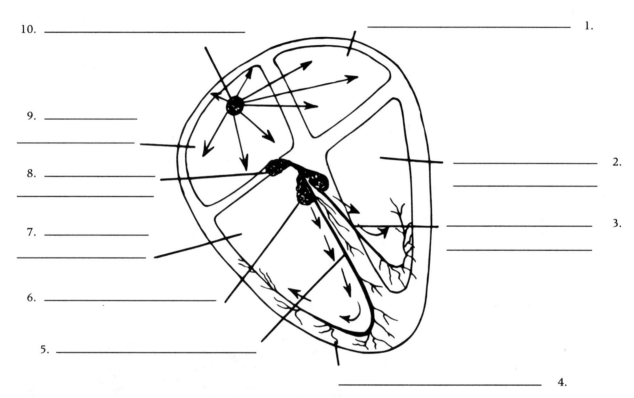

10. _____              _____ 1.

9. _____

8. _____              _____ 2.

7. _____              _____ 3.

6. _____

5. _____              _____ 4.

**Figure 55-1**

Left bundle branch                          Left atrium.

### PART B. DRUG EFFECT ON CARDIAC PHYSIOLOGY

Use the number associated with the correct answer from Part A of this exercise to correctly answer the following completion exercise.

1. *Bretylium* is used for treating serious refractory arrhythmias originating in this heart chamber:

   _____.

2. *Verapamil,* a calcium channel blocker, is used to treat supraventricular tachycardia and atrial

   fibrillation and flutter because it slows the electrical impulses originating in the _____

   and because it slows conduction through the _____.

3. *Atropine* is the drug of choice for heart block because it improves conduction first through this part of the heart, _____, and increases conduction through these parts of the heart: _____, _____, _____, _____, and _____.

4. *Disopyramide* (Norpace), which is given orally to adults to treat ventricular tachyarrhythmias, works by reducing automaticity in the _____ node, slowing conduction through the _____ node, and prolonging the refractory period.

## Arrhythmias analysis exercise

Select the appropriate term from the accompanying list to identify each of the following common arrhythmias and a drug that might be ordered to treat the arrhythmia.

Digoxin (Lanoxin)                        Premature ventricular contractions
Atropine                                 Sinus bradycardia
Atrial fibrillation                      Adenosine (Adenocard)
Supraventricular tachycardia             Lidocaine (Xylocaine)

1. Arrhythmia _____     Treatment _____

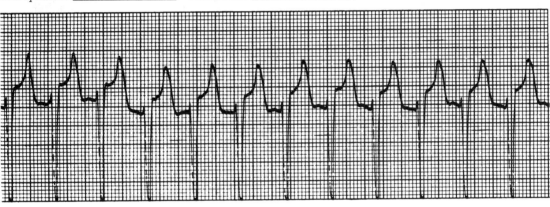

2. Arrhythmia _____     Treatment _____

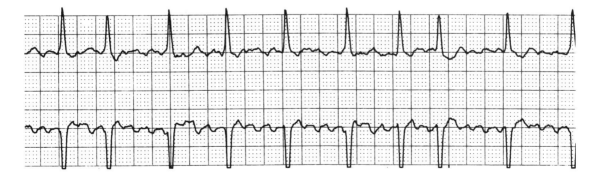

3. Arrhythmia _____ Treatment _____

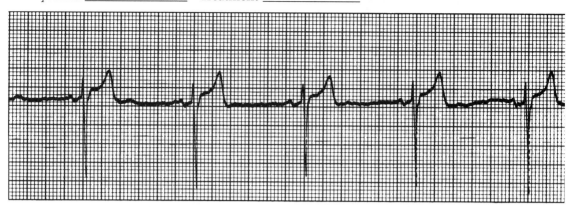

4. Arrhythmia _____ Treatment _____

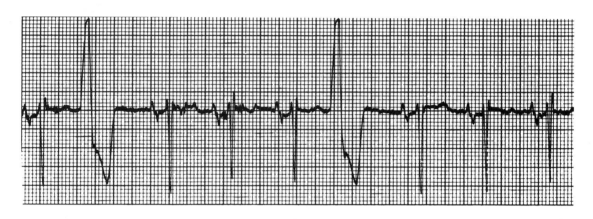

## Review questions

1. Mr. T. is started on quinidine 200 mg PO q6h. Which of the following would be an adverse effect of the quinidine therapy?

   a. Seizures.
   b. Rash.

   c. Headache.
   d. Diarrhea.

2. Which of the following behaviors by Mrs. C., who is taking propranolol (Inderal), indicates that your teaching has been successful? Mrs. C.

   a. increases her fluid intake to 3000 cc/day.
   b. reports a weight gain of over 2 lbs. in 1 week.

   c. takes multivitamins daily.
   d. takes her pulse once a week.

3. Side effects of lidocaine (Xylocaine) therapy that the nurse should be observing for include

   a. dysphagia.
   b. disorientation.

   c. excessive bruising.
   d. tinnitus.

4. After you have administered a bolus of lidocaine (Xylocaine), you will run a continuous infusion at the following rate:

   a. 0.25–0.75 mg/min.
   b. 10–20 mcg/min.

   c. 1–4 mg/min.
   d. 6–8 mg/min.

5. Identify which of the following drugs may be used to terminate supraventricular tachycardia:

    a. Lidocaine (Xylocaine).
    b. Flecainide (Tambocor).

    c. Esmolol (Brevibloc).
    d. Bretylium (Bretylol).

6. Persons taking a beta adrenergic blockers such as propranolol (Inderal) for their antiarrhythmic effect should be observed for

    a. tachycardia.
    b. hypertension.

    c. asthma.
    d. diarrhea.

7. The cardiac antiarrhythmic that can cause gingival hyperplasia is

    a. phenytoin (Dilantin).
    b. propranolol (Inderal).

    c. lidocaine (Xylocaine).
    d. esomolol (Brevibloc).

8. Mr. J. is being sent home on disopyramide (Norpace) for atrial fibrillation. He asks you why he must continue to take this drug. Your best response should be that atrial fibrillation

    a. can lead to the formation of thrombi in the atria.
    b. will result in the ventricles beating independently.

    c. may result in death.
    d. can cause edema in the extremities.

9. The physician plans on treating Mrs. H., who has atrial fibrillation, with quinidine. Prior to initiating treatment with quinidine, Mrs. H. should be taught to

    a. report ankle edema to her physician.
    b. check her blood pressure daily.

    c. contact her physician if her urine turns pink.
    d. monitor her blood sugars daily.

10. Which of the following statements by Mrs. G. would lead you to believe that she has a good understanding of the teaching that you have done regarding quinidine?

    a. "I will take the medication with citrus juice."
    b. "I will increase the fiber in my diet."

    c. "I will take the medication with meals."
    d. "I will limit my salt intake."

11. Identify which of the following drugs is used to terminate premature ventricular contractions:

    a. Propranolol (Inderal).
    b. Adenosine (Adenocard).

    c. Verapamil (Calan).
    d. Lidocaine (Xylocaine).

12. A factor that would necessitate that the dosage of disopyramide (Norpace) be reduced includes

    a. immobility.
    b. hypertension.

    c. renal impairment.
    d. chronic diarrhea.

## Critical thinking case study

Mr. J., a 56-year-old male weighing 195 lbs., is admitted to your unit with a diagnosis of myocardial infarction. You have standing orders in ICU that permit the use of lidocaine (Xylocaine) for treatment of 6 or more PVCs per minute.

1. Identify how much lidocaine (Xylocaine) you will administer as a bolus and how much you will give him as a maintenance infusion.

Mr. J. continues to have multifocal PVCs that are uncontrolled by lidocaine (Xylocaine).

2.  Discuss alternatives to the present treatment and your nursing responsibilities.

Mr. J.'s PVCs have resolved, and you are preparing to send him to the cardiac catheterization lab. His EKG shows a PR interval of 0.24 seconds. His heart rate is 60 and BP 106/68.

3.  It is time for Mr. J.'s propranolol (Inderal). In light of your observations, discuss what your actions will be.

Mr. J. is preparing for discharge and expresses concerns about resuming an active sex life and asks if the propranolol (Inderal) will affect it. (The student may need to use additional sources to answer this question.)

4.  Discuss your response to Mr. J.

# CHAPTER 56

# Antianginal Drugs

## Complete the following sentences

1. Nitrates work by reducing _____
   _____ and decreasing
   _____, which decreases
   _____ and _____. Nitrates increase blood
   _____ and lower _____.

2. Beta blockers reduce _____ and _____,
   _____, _____, and _____.

3. Calcium channel blockers dilate _____ and _____, decrease
   _____, and the conduction system is depressed.

4. Persons who have angina should avoid _____, _____, and
   _____.

5. Lifestyle changes that will help angina include _____, _____,
   and exercise.

6. Persons experiencing angina may take nitroglycerin, one every _____ minutes for a maximum of
   _____ doses. If the pain is unrelieved they should _____.

7. Adverse effects from nitroglycerin include _____, _____, and
   _____.

8. A person receiving beta blockers should be observed for _____, _____,
   _____, and _____.

9. Indicate side effects from administration of calcium channel blockers by placing an *X* next to the
   following:
   a. congestive heart failure _____.          e. anorexia _____.
   b. headache _____.                           f. confusion _____.
   c. diarrhea _____.                            g. nausea _____.
   d. weakness _____.

10. If dizziness occurs after the administration of antianginals, the client should
    _____ and _____.

## Matching exercise: terms and concepts

_____ 1. A drug used for the long-term treatment of chronic stable angina.

_____ 2. A calcium channel blocker used for angina and hypertension.

_____ 3. A drug used for the treatment of supraventricular tachycardias.

_____ 4. Onset of action of this drug is 1–3 minutes.

_____ 5. A common adverse effect of antianginal drugs.

_____ 6. This group of drugs is contraindicated in persons with congestive heart failure.

_____ 7. A beta adrenergic blocker given to prevent exercise-induced tachycardias.

_____ 8. This group of drugs, when administered with antianginals, will decrease their effects.

_____ 9. Tachycardia may occur with administration of this drug.

_____ 10. This drug, when given with antianginals, will increase their effects.

A. Nitroglycerin (Nitro-Bid).

B. Nicardipine (Cardene).

C. Anticholinergic drugs.

D. Hypertension.

E. Erythrityl tetranitrate (Cardilate).

F. Nifedipine (Procardia).

G. Verapamil (Calan).

H. Beta adrenergic blockers.

I. Hypotension.

J. Calcium channel blockers.

K. Propranolol (Inderal).

L. Cimetidine (Tagamet).

## Review questions

1. Mr. J., who has recently started taking nitroglycerin, complains of a headache. Your best response would be:
   a. "As your body becomes accustomed to the medication, the headaches will subside."
   b. "You will have to learn to live with the headaches."
   c. "In a few days the headaches will be gone."
   d. "The headaches are a sign that the medication is working; if you don't have a headache contact your physician."

2. Mr. J. is admitted with uncontrolled angina. He is currently taking nitroglycerin (Nitro-Bid). His physician adds nifedipine (Procardia) to his medication regimen. You should observe for
   a. hypokalemia.
   b. decreased urinary output.
   c. bradycardia.
   d. hypotension.

3. When doing the initial assessment on Mr. P., you discover that he has the following conditions. Which of the following conditions would necessitate that beta adrenergic blocking agents be administered with caution?
   a. Migraine headaches.
   b. Hypertension.
   c. Congestive heart failure.
   d. Tachycardia.

4. Which of the following statements by Mrs. M. would indicate that she has an adequate understanding of how nitroglycerin is to be administered?
   a. "Once I get a headache I know a therapeutic drug level has been reached and I will take no more medication."
   b. "I can take up to 3 tablets at 5-minute intervals."
   c. "I can take as much nitroglycerin as I need because it is not habit forming."
   d. "If I become dizzy after taking nitroglycerin, I should stop taking the medicine."

5. Beta adrenergic blockers help to control angina but may cause a(an)
   a. increased blood pressure.
   b. reduction in the force of contraction of the heart.
   c. increased oxygen consumption.
   d. reduced activity tolerance.

6. Your client can expect relief of chest pain when she takes sublingual nitroglycerin within
   a. 1–2 minutes.
   b. 5–10 minutes.
   c. 15–20 minutes.
   d. 30–60 minutes.

7. When instructing Mr. B. about nitroglycerin patches, you should tell him that the advantage of the patch is that
   a. it only has to be administered once a week.
   b. it is more effective in treating angina.
   c. it has a longer duration of action.
   d. it is faster acting than the tablets.

8. You are preparing Mr. P. for discharge after he has been diagnosed with angina. Which statement by Mr. P. leads you to believe that he has understood your discharge teaching?
   a. "I will not exercise because it will precipitate angina."
   b. "As long as I take the medicine I need to make no changes in my lifestyle."
   c. "There is no correlation between my hypertension and angina."
   d. "Heavy meals and cigarette smoking can precipitate angina."

9. Side effects that persons taking calcium channel blockers may experience include
   a. hypertension and tachycardia.
   b. headache and dizziness.
   c. flushing.
   d. nausea and diarrhea.

10. Persons receiving nifedipine (Procardia) should be assessed for
    a. ascites.
    b. asthma.
    c. peripheral edema.
    d. tetany.

## Critical thinking case study

Mr. D. comes to the emergency room complaining of severe chest pain. Three years ago his physician prescribed propranolol (Inderal) for hypertension which he stopped taking last year because of sexual dysfunction. The physician starts a nitroglycerin drop.

1. Identify what assessments you will make during the infusion of the nitroglycerin.

Once Mr. D. has stabilized he is started on diltiazem (Cardizem).

2. Explain the rationale for the choice of this drug to treat Mr. D.'s angina.

3. Identify the side effects of the drug that you will discuss with Mr. D.

Mr. D.'s physician also orders a nitroglycerin patch which is to be put on at 6 A.M. and taken off at 10 P.M.

4. Explain to the client why he is to use the patch in this way and what the potential side effects are.

# CHAPTER 57

# Drugs Used in Hypotension and Shock

## True or false

_____ 1. Alkalosis may decrease the effectiveness of dopamine (Intropin).

_____ 2. Dobutamine (Dobutrex) will decrease cardiac output.

_____ 3. When small doses of dopamine are administered, the client may experience hypotension.

_____ 4. Epinephrine (Adrenalin) can produce ventricular arrhythmias and reduce renal blood flow.

_____ 5. Isoproterenol (Isuprel) decreases the heart rate and increases diastolic blood pressure.

_____ 6. If extravasation of dopamine (Intropin) or levarterenol (Levophed) occurs, severe tissue damage can result.

_____ 7. Dopamine (Intropin), dobutamine (Dobutrex), and isoproterenol (Isuprel) can be administered orally or parenterally.

_____ 8. Vasopressors can increase oxygen consumption and produce myocardial ischemia.

_____ 9. Beta adrenergic blockers administered concurrently with vasopressors increase the effect of the vasopressor agent.

_____ 10. Adequate fluid therapy is necessary for dopamine (Intropin) to be effective.

## Complete the following sentences

1. Common symptoms of shock include _____ urinary output, _____ cardiac output, _____ orientation, seizures, cool extremities, and coma.

2. Drugs with alpha adrenergic activity increase _____ _____.

3. Drugs with beta adrenergic activity increase _____ and _____.

4. When treating someone for shock, you want to keep his or her blood pressure above _____, heart rate below 100, and urinary output above _____.

5. The drug of choice for treating extravasation is _____ (_____).

## Review questions

1. Vasopressor drugs are useful in treating
   a. postural hypotension.
   b. hypotension resulting from decreased cardiac output.
   c. hypotension secondary to anemia.
   d. hypotension secondary to anesthesia.

2. Mr. B. is admitted to ICU with a diagnosis of cardiogenic shock. Which one of the following should be reported?
   a. Temperature of 100.8°F.
   b. Nausea and vomiting.
   c. Urinary output of less than 30 cc/hr.
   d. Abdominal distention.

3. Because of the client's diagnosis of septic shock, which of the following nursing diagnoses would be a priority?
   a. Altered tissue perfusion.
   b. Activity intolerance.
   c. Social isolation.
   d. Altered bowel elimination.

4. Mr. H. is admitted with hypovolemic shock secondary to blood loss. Which of these nursing actions would take priority?
   a. Monitor intake and weight.
   b. Assess lung and bowel sounds.
   c. Check peripheral pulses and skin temperature.
   d. Check blood pressure and pulse.

5. Mr. G. is in your unit with a gunshot wound. His family is very concerned about him and questions why dobutamine (Dobutrex) is being used. Your best reply is:
   a. "We are giving this drug to increase Mr. G.'s heart rate and blood pressure."
   b. "This drug will improve Mr. G.'s condition."
   c. "This drug will increase the force of contraction of his heart and increase the blood supply to his vital organs."
   d. "We want to slow down Mr. G.'s heart rate and increase his blood pressure, and this drug will do that."

6. Mr. J. is started on an IV drip of dopamine (Intropin) for hypotension after open heart surgery. Identify what adverse effects you will be assessing for.
   a. Hypertension.
   b. Tachycardia.
   c. Bradycardia.
   d. Cyanosis.

7. Mr. P. is being treated for hypotension with dopamine (Intropin) and begins to complain of chest pain. Which of the following antianginal drugs would you question if it was ordered?
   a. Nitroglycerin (Nitro-Bid).
   b. Propranolol (Inderal).
   c. Diltiazem (Cardizem).
   d. Amyl nitrate (Vaporole).

8. J. has an IV of 200 mg of dopamine (Intropin) in 250 cc of 5 DW (800 µg/1/cc) If the physician wants J. to receive 400 µg/min, how fast will you run the IV? (Use micro-drip tubing, 1 cc = 60 gtts.)
   a. 15 gtts.
   b. 30 gtts.
   c. 60 gtts.
   d. 90 gtts.

9. If you note that levarterenol (Levophed) has extravasated, you should
   a. administer a beta adrenergic blocker.
   b. apply a tourniquet.
   c. apply ice and elevate the extremity.
   d. administer phentolamine (Regitine).

10. You have completed your teaching with Mr. P. who is being treated for congestive heart failure. Which of the following statements by Mr. P. leads you to believe he has understood the teaching you have done regarding dobutamine (Dobutrex)?

    a. "If I continue to have problems once I leave this unit, I can take dobutamine (Dobutrex) orally."
    b. "I know that they will be monitoring my pulse and blood pressure frequently."
    c. "I can expect severe headaches and I will not worry."
    d. "Nausea and vomiting are common so I will stick to clear liquids."

## Critical thinking case study

Mr. B. is admitted to ICU after a myocardial infarction. He is presently experiencing cardiogenic shock. The physician orders dopamine (Intropin) 200 mg in 250 ml of 5 DW. (Mr. B. weighs 220 lbs.)

1. Calculate the appropriate number of micrograms Mr. B. should be receiving per minute.

2. Identify the assessments you will perform and your rationale for each.

You have been unable to keep Mr. B.'s BP above 80/40 and his urinary output has dropped to 20 cc/hr. The physician decides to add dobutamine (Dobutrex).

3. Identify why Mr. B.'s physician is adding dobutamine (Dobutrex).

Mr. B. begins to experience chest pain. Nitroglycerin is added to his medication regime. Mr. B. has standing orders for $O_2$ and morphine 2 mg. (The student may want to use additional sources to answer this question.)

4.  Identify why Mr. B. is experiencing chest pain and list your nursing actions in order of priority.

# CHAPTER 58

# Antihypertensive Drugs

## Matching exercise: terms and concepts

### MATCH THE DRUG GROUP WITH ITS EFFECT.

_____ 1. Alpha$_1$ receptor blocking agent.

_____ 2. Alpha$_2$ receptor blocking agent.

_____ 3. Beta adrenergic blocking agent.

_____ 4. Calcium channel blocking agent.

_____ 5. Diuretics.

_____ 6. Vasodilators.

_____ 7. ACE inhibitor.

A. Blocks SNS impulses in the brain.

B. Decreases cardiac output and peripheral resistance.

C. Cause loss of sodium and water.

D. Cause dilation of blood vessels and decrease peripheral resistance; require concomitant use of a diuretic.

E. Dilates blood vessels and decreases peripheral resistance.

F. Decrease heart rate, force of the contraction, cardiac output, and renin release.

G. Blocks the enzyme that converts angiotensin I to angiotensin II.

### MATCH THE ANTIHYPERTENSIVE MEDICATION WITH THE GROUP IT IS INTENDED FOR.

_____ 1. Calcium channel blocker.

_____ 2. Vasodilators.

_____ 3. Thiazide diuretics.

_____ 4. Beta blockers.

_____ 5. ACE inhibitors.

A. May be used in children to treat hypertension.

B. Effective alone in white hypertensive clients.

C. Drugs of choice for persons with a high renin level.

D. Useful for clients who have angina and hypertension.

E. Should be used in combination with a diuretic.

## True or false

_____ 1. Beta adrenergic blockers should be used with caution for persons having congestive heart failure or asthma.

_____ 2. Oral contraceptives can increase the effect of antihypertensive medications.

_____ 3. Captopril (Capoten) should be administered with food.

_____ 4. Diazoxide (Hyperstat) is used in hypertensive crisis.

_____ 5. Thiazide diuretics can cause hyperglycemia, hyperuremia, and hypercalcemia in adults.

## Name that drug

_____  1.  Used to treat neonatal hypertension.

_____  2.  Used for hypertensive crisis; administered by rapid injection.

_____  3.  Commonly used as an IV drip after open heart surgery to maintain the blood pressure within normal limits.

_____  4.  A drug used for the treatment of mild hypertension that can cause potassium loss.

_____  5.  These are the drugs of choice for persons over 50 with high renin levels.

_____  6.  These drugs may be useful for persons who have angina and hypertension.

_____  7.  This group of drugs acts directly on the blood vessels to cause dilation.

_____  8.  Available in a skin patch that can be applied once a week.

_____  9.  A nonpharmacologic way of controlling blood pressure.

_____  10.  These drugs are effective in treating hypertension for persons with renal disease.

_____  11.  These antihypertensive medications produce hyperglycemia.

_____  12.  Depression is an adverse effect of this medication.

_____  13.  Abrupt withdrawal of this drug can cause a hypertensive crisis.

_____  14.  An ACE inhibitor used once daily for treatment of hypertension.

_____  15.  Antihypertensive medication used to treat chronic hypertension.

_____  16.  Insulin-dependent diabetics may have difficulty in controlling their blood sugars if they are placed on this drug to control their BP.

## Review questions

1.  The physician prescribes captopril (Capoten) for your client. You know that your teaching has been effective if your client says:

    a.  "I will limit my fluid intake to 1200 cc daily."

    b.  "I will make sure that I rise slowly from a supine position."

    c.  "I will take a laxative along with the antihypertensive medication."

    d.  "I will no longer be able to drive a car."

2.  Which of the following represents the most important outcome for Mr. J. who has recently been diagnosed with hypertension?

    a.  Verbalization of an understanding of his medical regime.

    b.  Confirmation that his prescriptions have been filled.

    c.  Evidence of a systolic BP above 100 and below 140.

    d.  Evidence of a pulse below 80.

3.  Mrs. H., who is being treated for hypertension, should be instructed to avoid

    a.  citrus fruits.

    b.  baked potatoes.

    c.  sandwich meats.

    d.  fish.

4. Which of the following statements by your client would indicate a good understanding of what you have taught her regarding hypertension?

   a. "If I think my blood pressure is high, I will take an extra pill."

   b. "When I no longer have headaches, I can stop taking the medication."

   c. "For relaxation I will soak in a hot tub."

   d. "If I feel dizzy, I will still take my medication and have my blood pressure checked."

5. Mrs. Y. is to be placed on reserpine (Serpasil). Prior to administration of this medication, the nurse will ask Mrs. Y. if she has a history of

   a. depression.

   b. glaucoma.

   c. diabetes mellitus.

   d. seizures.

6. Besides decreasing Mr. P.'s blood pressure, an expected outcome after the administration of propranolol (Inderal) is

   a. increased urinary output.

   b. decreased heart rate.

   c. increased heart rate.

   d. decreased urinary output.

7. Mrs. P. should be taught to expect the following side effects related to hydralazine (Apresoline) therapy:

   a. Sodium and water retention.

   b. Potassium loss.

   c. Blood dyscrasias.

   d. Constipation.

8. Persons experiencing hypertension and angina are best treated with

   a. beta adrenergic blockers.

   b. direct-acting vasodilators.

   c. alpha blocking agents.

   d. ganglionic blocking agents.

9. Angiotensin converting enzyme (ACE) inhibitors work by

   a. stimulating the release of renin.

   b. blocking the enzyme that converts angiotensin I to angiotensin II.

   c. increasing peripheral resistance.

   d. blocking SNS impulses in the brain.

10. Mr. Green is receiving propranolol (Inderal). He has the following complaints. Which one may be directly related to the Inderal?

   a. Headache.

   b. Chest pain.

   c. Palpitations.

   d. Nausea.

## Critical thinking case study

Your client M. is a 35-year-old black female race-car driver who weighs 200 lbs. and smokes two packages of cigarettes per day. Her doctor prescribes propranolol (Inderal) for her essential hypertension.

1. Identify what lifestyle changes would help M. lower her blood pressure.

2.  Identify the potential complications related to hypertension that you plan on discussing with M.

3.  Discuss the teaching you will do with M.

4.  Identify ways of promoting compliance.

Three years after her initial treatment for hypertension, M. is seen at the physician's office. Her BP is 180/90 and she has symptoms of chronic renal failure. The physician changes her medication to enalapril (Vasotec) and bumetanide (Bumex).

5.  Discuss why M.'s physician ordered two medications at this time.

# CHAPTER 59

# Diuretics

## Complete the following sentences

1. The nephron functions by three processes: _____, _____, and _____.

2. A minimum daily urine output of _____ is required to remove _____ of _____.

3. Most reabsorption occurs in the _____.

4. _____ promotes reabsorption of _____ from the distal tubules and collecting ducts.

5. _____, a hormone from the adrenal cortex, promotes _____ reabsorption and _____ loss.

6. In the proximal tubules _____, _____, _____, and _____ are secreted.

7. In the distal tubules _____, _____, and _____ are secreted.

8. Edema occurs because of _____, _____, and _____.

9. Diuretics are often used for persons with edema because they mobilize _____ by _____.

10. Diuretics are used for persons with hypertension because they decrease _____ and deplete _____, which may _____.

11. _____ are the most frequently prescribed diuretic agents. The diuretic effect occurs within _____ hours.

12. Potassium-sparing diuretics decrease the exchange of _____ for _____.
_____ is the major adverse effect.

13. Osmotic agents increase _____ (_____) which causes _____
to be pulled from extravascular sites into the _____. _____ (Osmitrol) has
many uses.

14. Prior to administering diuretics, the following blood values should be assessed because diuretics can
alter these values: _____, _____, _____,
_____, and _____.

15. Other assessments that the nurse should do when a person is receiving diuretics include measuring
_____, _____, _____, and
_____.

16. When diuretics are given with digoxin, there is an increased risk of _____
related to _____.

17. A normal serum potassium level is _____.

18. If hypokalemia should occur, it can be treated in the following ways: _____,
_____, _____ potassium _____,
_____, and _____.

19. Hypokalemia can produce the following symptoms: _____,
_____, _____, _____, _____,
_____, _____, _____, and
_____.

## True or false

_____ 1. Hypoglycemia is a common side effect that can be reversed when diuretic therapy is discontinued.

_____ 2. Hyperuricemia can cause gout in persons taking diuretics.

_____ 3. Loop diuretics, when administered rapidly, can cause transient hearing loss.

_____ 4. When loop diuretics are administered with aminoglycosides, the effect of the diuretic is decreased.

_____ 5. Hypernatremia, hypermagnesemia, and hyperchloremia are common with the long-term use of diuretics.

## The nephron

Fill in the blanks in Figure 59-1 with the following terms:

Descending limb of loop of Henle       Glomerulus
Bowman's capsule       Loop of Henle
Collecting tubule       Distal tubule
Efferent arteriole       Ascending limb of loop of Henle
Afferent arteriole       Proximal tubule

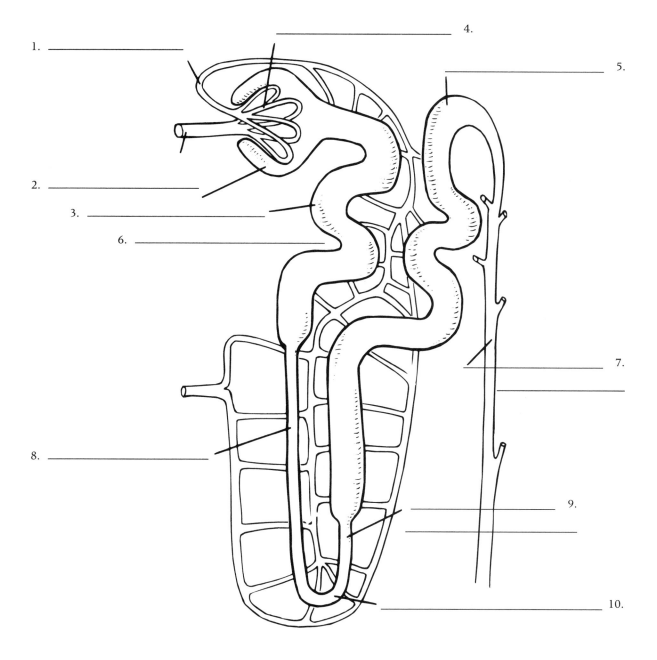

**Figure 59-1**

## Review questions

1. Diuretics are used to treat edema which occurs because of
   a. decreased capillary permeability.
   b. decreased capillary hydrostatic pressure.
   c. decreased plasma osmotic pressure.
   d. decreased serum sodium levels.

2. When loop diuretics are administered intravenously, you can expect to see a response to the medication in
   a. 5 minutes.
   b. 15 to 20 minutes.
   c. 30 to 60 minutes.
   d. 2 hours.

3. Mrs. J. is an insulin-dependent diabetic. Prior to administering hydrochlorothiazide (Hydrodiuril) you should inform her that
   a. her insulin dose may need to be increased.
   b. her insulin dose may need to be decreased.
   c. she will need to check her blood sugar four times a day.
   d. she will need to have a creatinine clearance done once a month.

4. When evaluating your client for adverse effects of hydrochlorothiazide (Hydrodiuril), which of the following lab values would be significant?
   a. Elevated uric acid levels.
   b. Reduced blood urea nitrogen levels.
   c. A serum potassium level of 5.0 mEq/liter.
   d. A blood sugar of 70.

5. Which of the following statements by your client makes you believe that she understands your teaching about diuretics?
   a. "I will weigh myself once a week and report any changes."
   b. "I will no longer have to watch what I eat."
   c. "If my leg gets swollen again, I'll just take 2 pills instead of 1."
   d. "I will take my medication at night."

6. Mr. C. is admitted and the physician draws a serum potassium. Which of the following values is within the normal range?
   a. 2.1–3.4 mEq/liter.
   b. 3.5–5.0 mEq/liter.
   c. 5.1–6.5 mEq/liter.
   d. 6.6–7.9 mEq/liter.

7. Mrs. B. is started on furosemide (Lasix) 40 mg daily. You will check her lab values on a regular basis because you know a side effect of this medication is
   a. hyperchloremia.
   b. hyponatremia.
   c. hyperkalemia.
   d. hypophosphatemia.

8. When administering intravenous furosemide (Lasix), you will administer it slowly because if it is administered rapidly, it can cause
   a. renal failure.
   b. respiratory distress.
   c. blindness.
   d. hearing loss.

9. Spironolactone (Aldactone) should not be administered to persons with
   a. diabetes mellitus.
   b. elevated serum potassium levels.
   c. elevated serum sodium levels.
   d. hypertension.

10. Which of the following is an osmotic diuretic?
    a. Spironolactone (Aldactone).
    b. Bumetanide (Bumex).
    c. Mannitol (Osmitrol).
    d. Ethacrynic (Edecrin).

## Critical thinking case study

Mr. P., a 69-year-old, is admitted with acute congestive heart failure. His physician orders digoxin (Lanoxin) 0.25 mg, furosemide (Lasix) 20 mg b.i.d., and spironolactone (Aldactone) 25 mg b.i.d.

1. Discuss why Mr. P.'s physician ordered these medications.

2. Identify what you should be assessing for (including lab values).

Three days after admission, Mr. P. has lost 10 lbs. When you go in to his room to do his morning assessment, you find that he is confused.

3. Identify your nursing actions.

# CHAPTER 60

# Anticoagulant, Antiplatelet, and Thrombolytic Agents

## Complete the chart

| Drug | Mechanism of Action | Antidote | Administration | Lab Test and Onset of Action |
|------|---------------------|----------|----------------|------------------------------|
| Heparin | | | | |
| Warfarin sodium (Coumadin) | | | | |
| Aspirin | | | | |
| Streptokinase | | | | |

## Drug interactions

Indicate whether the following drugs increase or decrease the effects of Coumadin:

1. Tetracycline  _____
2. Clofibrate  _____
3. Cholestyramine  _____
4. Maalox  _____
5. Cimetidine  _____

6. Estrogen  _____
7. Amitriptyline  _____
8. Synthroid  _____
9. Lasix  _____
10. Alcohol  _____

## Review questions

1. The effects of warfarin sodium (Coumadin) are monitored by the following lab test:

   a. CBC.                                c. PT.
   b. APTT.                               d. BUN.

2. Bleeding resulting from the administration of heparin should be treated with

   a. vitamin E.                          c. protamine sulfate.
   b. vitamin K.                          d. calcium gluconate.

3. You know that your client needs additional teaching regarding anticoagulants if he states:

   a. "I will carry a Medic Alert card with me."    c. "I will use aspirin for arthritis pain."
   b. "I will report to the lab once a month."      d. "I will use an electric razor."

4. Persons taking Coumadin should minimize foods high in vitamin K, including

   a. eggs.                               c. citrus fruits.
   b. milk.                               d. fish.

5. You know that your teaching about Coumadin is successful if your client states:

   a. "If I miss a dose, I will take 2 pills       c. "I will increase the dark-green leafy
      the next day."                                  vegetables in my diet."
   b. "I will not drink alcoholic beverages."      d. "I can still take over-the-counter medi-
                                                      cations if I have a cold."

6. Mr. G., who is receiving Coumadin, has blood in his urinary drainage bag this morning. After reporting her observations to the physician, the nurse will administer

   a. Amicar.                             c. protamine sulfate.
   b. platelets.                          d. vitamin K.

7. Mr. L., who is receiving streptokinase for a myocardial infarction, passes a large amount of blood with his stool. The nurse will notify the physician and expect to

   a. reduce the streptokinase and        c. reduce the streptokinase and
      administer vitamin K.                   administer heparin.
   b. stop the streptokinase and administer   d. stop the streptokinase and
      protamine sulfate.                      administer Amicar.

8. Mr. P. is admitted with thrombophlebitis and is started on heparin. You know that Mr. P. has a good understanding of why heparin is being used if he states that heparin will

   a. inhibit the formation of additional clots.   c. prevent the blood from clotting.
   b. eliminate certain clotting factors.          d. dissolve the clot.

9. Mrs. C. is receiving a continuous drip of heparin 1000 units/hr. The nurse should

   a. avoid intramuscular injections.     c. take hourly urinary outputs.
   b. assess Mrs. C. for symptoms of      d. take hourly vital signs.
      respiratory depression.

10. Miss H. is receiving subcutaneous heparin. When the nurse administers the heparin, he or she should

    a. apply pressure to the injection site.   c. gently massage the site after the injection.
    b. insert the needle at a 45° angle.       d. use the Z track method.

## Critical thinking case study

M., a 25-year-old female, has been hospitalized with a fractured femur after a motor vehicle accident. M. weighs 200 lbs., smokes one package of cigarettes per day, and is taking birth control pills and Diabeta. M.'s BP is 180/90, pulse 90, respirations 24 when she is admitted. The physician orders heparin 5,000 units SC q12h.

1. Identify what assessments you would do before you administer the heparin.

During the night, M. becomes short of breath and complains of chest pain. (Additional sources will be necessary to answer this question.)

2. Identify and prioritize your nursing actions.

The physician diagnoses M. with a pulmonary embolism and starts M. on a continuous infusion of heparin (1000 units/hr).

3. Discuss why M. was at high risk for developing pulmonary embolism.

M. is started on warfarin (Coumadin) while she is still receiving heparin.

4.  Discuss why the two anticoagulants are being given together.

5.  Identify how the dosage of Coumadin is determined.

6.  Describe the teaching you will do with M. to prepare her for discharge.

# CHAPTER 61

# Antilipemics and Peripheral Vasodilators

## Matching exercise: terms and concepts

Match the drug with its side effects.

_____ 1. Cholestyramine (Questran).

_____ 2. Gemfibrozil (Lopid).

_____ 3. Lovastatin (Mevacor).

_____ 4. Nicotinic acid (Niacin).

_____ 5. Pentoxifylline (Trental).

_____ 6. Isoxsuprine (Vasodilan).

A. Flushing of head and neck.

B. Weakness, muscle cramps, increased angina.

C. Constipation.

D. Headache, skin rash, pruritus.

E. Tachycardia, hypotension, dizziness.

F. Dyspepsia, nausea, vomiting.

## True or false

_____ 1. Diet and exercise are the first line of treatment for hyperlipoproteinemia.

_____ 2. Cholestyramine (Questran) decreases absorption of many drugs.

_____ 3. Isoxsuprine hydrochloride (Vasodilan) may cause hypertension and bradycardia.

_____ 4. Nylidrin hydrochloride (Arlidin) may cause flushing of the head and neck.

_____ 5. Bile acid–sequestering agents should be taken in dry form to prevent esophageal irritation.

_____ 6. Discharge teaching of clients receiving cholestyramine (Questran) should include information on preventing constipation.

_____ 7. Probucol (Lorelco) should be administered on an empty stomach.

_____ 8. Persons taking niacin may experience headaches and blurred vision.

_____ 9. A person taking probucol (Lorelco) can expect that his cholesterol will be lowered in 1–3 months.

_____ 10. If antilipemics fail to lower cholesterol in 2–3 months they should be discontinued.

## Review questions

1. Mr. S. is to be started on pentoxifylline (Trental) for his peripheral vascular disease. For which of the following sensitivities would pentoxifylline (Trental) be contraindicated?

   a. Shellfish

   b. Aged cheese.

   c. Alcohol.

   d. Caffeine.

2. Which one of the following statements by Mrs. G. leads you to believe that she understands the teaching that you have done regarding pentoxifylline (Trental)?
   a. "I will take the medication with meals."
   b. "I will increase the roughage in my diet."
   c. "I will weigh myself weekly."
   d. "I will have my blood pressure checked weekly."

3. Mrs. B., a diabetic with elevated cholesterol, is receiving gemfibrozil (Lopid) and should be taught to report the following adverse effects of the medication to her physician:
   a. Dizziness.
   b. Headaches.
   c. Chest pain.
   d. Diplopia.

4. Mrs. J. is started on an antilipemic. Which of the following statements would lead you to believe that she needs additional teaching?
   a. "I will eat foods high in fiber."
   b. "I know I must work on losing weight and quitting smoking."
   c. "I will exercise 20 minutes daily."
   d. "Now that I am taking this medication, I can eat whatever I want."

5. Papaverine (Pavabid) is ordered for Mrs. K., who has diabetes mellitus, hypertension, and peripheral vascular disease, to
   a. treat peripheral ischemia associated with vasospasm.
   b. stop the atherosclerotic changes.
   c. produce vasoconstriction of the vascular smooth muscle.
   d. prevent the development of a thrombus.

6. Because of the possible adverse effects associated with lovastatin (Mevacor), the nurse should schedule Mr. B. for which of the following?
   a. Monthly $T_3$ and $T_4$ levels.
   b. Liver function studies every 4–6 weeks.
   c. Monthly ECGs.
   d. Weekly WBCs.

7. Before Mrs. H. is started on niacin, she should be given all of the following instructions *except*
   a. You may experience nausea and dyspepsia from this medication.
   b. If you experience flushing of the head and neck, don't be alarmed; there is nothing you can do for it.
   c. Skin rashes and pruritus are common side effects of this drug.
   d. You may experience hypotension and dizziness so move slowly from a sitting to a standing position.

8. Which of the following statements is true regarding antilipemics?
   a. Each drug is specific for one type of hyperlipemia.
   b. All antilipemic drugs are effective against all types of hyperlipidemia.
   c. Each drug is recommended for the treatment of special types of hyperlipidemia.
   d. No antilipemic drug will also lower triglycerides.

9. A disease that a person taking clofibrate (Atromid-S) should be evaluated for is
   a. diabetes mellitus.
   b. anemia.
   c. cholelithiasis.
   d. colitis.

10. A bile acid–sequestering agent may cause a deficiency of fat-soluble vitamins. Identify which one of the following medications is a bile acid–sequestering agent:
    a. Cholestyramine (Questran).
    b. Clofibrate (Atromid-S).
    c. Gemfibrozil (Lopid).
    d. Lovastatin (Mevacor).

## Critical thinking case study

Mr. J., a 55-year-old male, is admitted with leg ulcers and peripheral edema secondary to peripheral vascular disease. He is being evaluated for a bypass graft. His physician orders isoxsuprine hydrochloride (Vasodilan) 20 mg q.i.d. (Students may need to use additional sources to answer the questions below.)

1. Identify the assessments you will perform when Mr. J. is initially admitted and your rationale for each.

After several doses of Vasodilan, you check Mr. J.'s vital signs and find that his pulse is 98 and BP 80/60. He is complaining of dizziness and has palpable peripheral pulses.

2. Identify and prioritize your nursing actions.

Mr. J.'s physician changes his medication to pentoxifylline (Trental) and nylidrin (Arlidin).

3. Discuss the discharge teaching that you will do with Mr. J.

# SECTION X

# Drugs Affecting the Digestive System

---

## CHAPTER 62

## Physiology of the Digestive System

---

## Matching exercise: terms and concepts

_____ 1. Propels food through the GI tract.

_____ 2. Stimulation of this system increases motility and secretions.

_____ 3. This system shunts blood away from the digestive tract.

_____ 4. Muscular fibrous tube whose main function is to convey food to the stomach.

_____ 5. Secretes intrinsic factor.

_____ 6. The sphincter at the beginning of the duodenum.

_____ 7. When the stomach normally empties.

_____ 8. A hormone produced by the duodenal mucosa that inhibits gastric secretion and motility.

_____ 9. The first 10–12 inches of the small intestine.

_____ 10. The portion of the small intestine that opens into the cecum.

_____ 11. The portion of the large intestine that absorbs water.

_____ 12. This organ secretes enzymes that are necessary for digestion of carbohydrates, proteins, and fats.

_____ 13. Releases bile when fats are present in the duodenum.

_____ 14. This organ synthesizes bile, serum albumin and globulin, prothrombin, fibrinogen, other blood coagulation factors, and urea.

_____ 15. Provides the acid medium to promote pepsin activity.

A. Stomach.

B. Enterogastrone.

C. Duodenum.

D. Peristalsis.

E. Parasympathetic nervous system.

F. Sympathetic nervous system.

G. Esophagus.

H. Trachea.

I. Pyloric.

J. Cardiac.

K. 4 hours.

L. 2 hours.

M. Ileum.

N. Cecum.

O. Pancreas.

P. Gall bladder.

Q. Liver.

R. Hydrochloric acid.

S. Bile.

T. Gastrin.

## Review questions

1.  This organ regulates glucose metabolism and blood sugar levels:
    a.  Liver.
    b.  Gall bladder.
    c.  Pancreas.
    d.  Small intestine.

2.  This substance is required for digestion and absorption of fats and fat-soluble vitamins:
    a.  Hydrochloric acid.
    b.  Bile.
    c.  Pancreatic juice.
    d.  Gastric juice.

3.  When liver functioning is impaired, toxic levels of this substance can build up and result in coma or death:
    a.  Ammonia.
    b.  Hormones.
    c.  Glucose.
    d.  Bilirubin.

4.  Which of the following organs secretes the intrinsic factor that is necessary for the absorption of vitamin $B_{12}$?
    a.  Pancreas.
    b.  Liver.
    c.  Gall bladder.
    d.  Stomach.

5.  The bile duct empties into the
    a.  duodenum.
    b.  jejunum.
    c.  ileum.
    d.  cecum.

6.  This portion of the intestine is where water is absorbed:
    a.  Duodenum.
    b.  Jejunum.
    c.  Ileum.
    d.  Cecum.

7.  When mucus secretion is absent, the following will occur:
    a.  Diarrhea.
    b.  Ulceration.
    c.  Constipation.
    d.  Distention.

8.  Saliva has a pH of:
    a.  2 to 3.
    b.  4 to 5.
    c.  6 to 7.
    d.  8 or above.

9.  Stimulation of the sympathetic nervous system will
    a.  increase peristalsis.
    b.  decrease peristalsis.
    c.  have no impact on peristalsis.

10. The following hormone is released when fats are present in the duodenum:
    a.  Enterogastrone.
    b.  Gastrin.
    c.  Pepsin.
    d.  Lipase.

# CHAPTER 63

# Drugs Used in Peptic Ulcer Disease

## Matching exercise: terms and concepts

_____ 1. Prevent the release of gastric acid into the stomach lumen.

_____ 2. Inhibit gastric acid secretion.

_____ 3. Increase mucus production.

_____ 4. Used with other agents to further reduce gastric acid secretion.

_____ 5. React with hydrochloric acid in the stomach to raise the pH.

_____ 6. Large doses are required; the drugs cause constipation, clients may develop hypophosphatemia.

_____ 7. High neutralizing capacity; cause diarrhea and hypermagnesemia.

_____ 8. Rapid onset of action; may cause alkalosis.

_____ 9. Aluminum-based antacid used to lower serum phosphate levels.

_____ 10. An antiflatulent.

A. Anticholinergic agents.

B. Gastric acid pump inhibitors.

C. Histamine–2 receptor blocking agents.

D. Prostaglandins.

E. Antacids.

F. Calcium compounds.

G. Amphogel.

H. Sodium bicarbonate.

I. Magnesium compounds.

J. Simethicone (Mylicon).

## True or false

_____ 1. Alcohol and caffeine can cause gastric irritation.

_____ 2. Protein and calcium in milk decrease secretion of gastric acid.

_____ 3. Ulcers are usually treated with sucralfate (Carafate) for 2–4 weeks.

_____ 4. Antacids increase the effectiveness of cimetidine (Tagamet) and sucralfate (Carafate).

_____ 5. Avoiding highly spiced and gas-forming foods prevents ulcer formation.

## Complete the following sentences

1. Besides peptic ulcer disease, antacids are also used in the treatment of _____, _____, and _____.

2. Omeprazole (Prilosec) inhibits gastric acid secretion by preventing the release of _____ into the stomach lumen.

3. Cimetidine (Tagamet) decreases _____ and _____ of gastric juices.

4. Ranitidine (Zantac) is more _____ than cimetidine (Tagamet) and has fewer _____.

5. Famotidine (_____) and nizatidine (_____) are also used to treat ulcers but are less likely to cause _____ and _____.

6. Misoprostol (_____) is indicated for clients with a high risk of _____.

7. Sucralfate (_____) adheres to the _____ and forms a protective _____ to promote _____.

8. Risk factors for peptic ulcer disease include:

   a. _____.
   b. _____.
   c. _____.
   d. _____.
   e. _____.
   f. _____.

## Matching exercise: terms and concepts

Match the following drugs that interact with cimetidine (Tagamet) with their classification.

_____ 1. Antiarrhythmics.

_____ 2. Anticoagulants.

_____ 3. Benzodiazepine antianxiety or hypnotic agents.

_____ 4. Beta adrenergic blocking agents.

_____ 5. Bronchodilator.

_____ 6. Calcium channel blocker.

_____ 7. Tricyclic antidepressants.

_____ 8. Anticonvulsants.

A. Carbamazepine, phenytoin.

B. Verapamil.

C. Alprazolam, chlordiazepoxide, diazepam, flurazepam, triazolam.

D. Lidocaine, quinidine.

E. Theophylline.

F. Warfarin.

G. Labetalol, metoprolol, propranolol.

H. Amitriptyline.

# Crossword puzzle

**Across**

1. A synthetic form of prostaglandin E: helpful to counter gastric acid caused by NSAIDs.
4. Antacids with high _____ content should be contraindicated in edematous states.
9. _____ carbonate overuse may cause hypercalcemia.
10. Calcium antacids are rarely used for peptic ulcers since they can cause _____ of gastric acid.

**Down**

2. This type of antacid can cause abortion.
3. It is important that a patient be matched with an antacid that has this quality.
5. A drug that can prevent the development of stress ulcers.
6. Antacids containing this element may cause constipation.
7. A gastric-acid-inhibiting drug in a time-release capsule.
8. The only approved cytoprotective drug: binds to ulcerated mucosa.

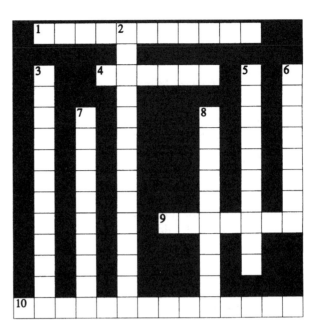

# Review questions

1. A synthetic prostaglandin used for prevention of peptic ulcers is
   a. misoprostol (Cytotec).
   b. famotidine (Pepcid).
   c. sucralfate (Carafate).
   d. cimetidine (Tagamet).

2. The ideal time to administer sucralfate (Carafate) is
   a. 1 hour after meals.
   b. 1 hour before meals and h.s.
   c. 30 minutes before meals with milk.
   d. with meals.

3. The following is the antacid of choice for persons with renal disease:
   a. Maalox.
   b. Amphojel.
   c. Di-Gel.
   d. Mylanta.

4. Which of the following statements by your client would lead you to believe that he needs further instruction about the medications he is taking for his peptic ulcer disease?
   a. "I will take the antacids an hour before meals with the sucralfate (Carafate)."
   b. "I will chew my antacid tablets before swallowing them."
   c. "I will take cimetidine (Tagamet) with meals."
   d. "I will shake the Maalox each time before I use it."

5. Histamine-2 receptor blockers work by
   a. increasing mucus production in the gastric mucosa.
   b. preventing the release of gastric acid into the stomach lumen.
   c. neutralizing gastric acid.
   d. inhibiting gastric acid secretion.

6. Mrs. H., a 79-year-old female with peptic ulcer disease, has become confused on the third day she is in the hospital. Upon reviewing her medication record, you notice that one of the following medications can cause confusion:

   a. sucralfate (Carafate).

   b. omeprazole (Prilosec).

   c. misoprostol (Cytotec).

   d. cimetidine (Tagamet).

7. Miss J., a 21-year-old nursing student, is admitted to your unit with a diagnosis of peptic ulcer disease. Which of the following could be a contributing factor to her developing the disease?

   a. She is female and 21 years of age.

   b. She takes birth control pills.

   c. She smokes a package of cigarettes a day.

   d. She is of Italian descent.

8. Miss J., with peptic ulcer disease, is to be discharged. What information do you include in your discharge teaching?

   a. Drink plenty of milk.

   b. Avoid alcohol and caffeine.

   c. Spicy foods should have no effect on your ulcer.

   d. You can take antacids as frequently as you would like; they have no side effects.

9. Persons taking calcium compounds to neutralize stomach acid should be assessed for

   a. constipation.

   b. hyperphosphatemia.

   c. hypomagnesemia.

   d. diarrhea.

10. Mrs. H. is having a great deal of flatulence after her surgery. Which of the following medications would be most helpful to her?

    a. Omeprazole (Prilosec).

    b. Gelusil.

    c. Mylanta.

    d. Simethicone (Mylicon).

## Critical thinking case study

Mr. J. is admitted with a duodenal ulcer because he is actively bleeding. The physician starts him on cimetidine (Tagamet).

1. Identify why Tagamet is ordered for Mr. J.

2. If 300 mg of Tagamet in 100 ml of 5 DW is to infuse over 20 minutes using macrodrip tubing (10 gtts. = 1 ml), how many drops per minute will you run the IV?

3.  Identify the adverse reactions from the Tagamet you will be observing for.

Mr. J. is no longer bleeding and the physician starts him on sucralfate (Carafate).

4.  Identify what you will be observing for.

5.  Identify what foods should be avoided in peptic ulcer disease and explain why.

6.  Discuss the instructions you will give Mr. J. prior to discharge.

# CHAPTER 64

# Laxatives and Cathartics

## Matching exercise: terms and concepts

_____ 1. These substances swell and become gel-like and stimulate peristalsis and defecation.

_____ 2. This laxative decreases the surface tension of the fecal mass, allowing water to penetrate into the stool.

_____ 3. These substances increase osmotic pressure in the intestinal lumen, causing water to be retained.

_____ 4. These drugs irritate the GI mucosa, pulling water into the bowel lumen.

_____ 5. Used as a suppository, it stimulates bowel evacuation by irritating the rectal mucosa.

_____ 6. This lubricates the intestine by retarding colonic absorption of fecal water.

_____ 7. A laxative that decreases the production of ammonia in the intestine.

_____ 8. A substance commonly mixed with Kayexalate to prevent constipation.

_____ 9. Used for fecal impaction.

_____ 10. An adverse effect of the administration of mineral oil.

_____ 11. Saline cathartics are contraindicated in renal disease because they may cause this

_____ 12. A product used to cleanse the bowel before surgery.

_____ 13. This saline cathartic is less likely to produce hyponatremia because it has sodium sulfate as its major component.

_____ 14. This laxative should be taken with a full glass of water.

_____ 15. Discoloration of urine may occur with this laxative.

A. Saline cathartics.

B. Mineral oil.

C. Sorbitol.

D. Stimulant cathartics.

E. Surfactant laxatives.

F. Bulk-forming laxatives.

G. Glycerin.

H. Lactulose (Chronulac).

I. Oil retention enema.

J. Decreased absorption of fat-soluble vitamins.

K. Anemia.

L. Hypermagnesmia.

M. Hyponatremia.

N. Magnesium citrate.

O. Polyethylene glycol-electrolyte solution (GoLYTELY).

P. Cascara sagrada (Cas-Exac).

Q. Psyllium preparations (Metamucil).

## Review questions

1. Which of the following drugs slow intestinal motility and put persons at risk for developing constipation?

   a. Tricyclic antidepressants.
   b. Thiazide diuretics.

   c. Calcium channel blockers.
   d. Thyroid preparations.

2. Mrs. J., who is taking a senna preparation (Senokot), calls you because she has noticed that her urine is a deep red and she thinks she is bleeding. Your best response would be:

   a. "Come in immediately and we will take a urine specimen."
   b. "Go directly to the emergency room and the doctor will meet you there."

   c. "The medication you are taking can color the urine different shades of red."
   d. "Drink 2000–3000 cc of acidic fluid every day and your urine will clear."

3. Which of the following statements by Mrs. H. leads you to believe that she has understood how to use bulk-forming laxatives?

   a. "I will mix the medication with 8 ounces of juice and follow it immediately by 8 ounces of juice."
   b. "I will mix the dry medication with applesauce."

   c. "I will use milk of magnesia in conjunction with this medication until I am having daily bowel movements."
   d. "I will decrease the roughage in my diet while I am using this medication."

4. An adverse effect of administration of stimulant cathartics is

   a. nausea.
   b. vomiting.

   c. diarrhea.
   d. lower GI bleeding.

5. Long-term administration of mineral oil can decrease the absorption of the following vitamins:

   a. Vitamin $B_{12}$.
   b. Vitamin C.

   c. Vitamin D.
   d. Vitamin $B_2$.

6. Long-term use of saline cathartics can produce the following electrolyte imbalance:

   a. Hypomagnesemia.
   b. Hyperkalemia.

   c. Hypochloremia.
   d. Hyperphosphatemia.

7. Which of the following ways of administering caster oil would make it more palatable?

   a. Heat it.
   b. Chill it.

   c. Dilute it with water.
   d. Flavor it with peppermint.

8. The safest and most effective way to treat constipation in children is with

   a. milk of magnesia.
   b. sorbitol.

   c. Dulcolax suppositories.
   d. glycerin suppositories.

9. Mr. J. is an alcoholic with chronic liver failure. Which of the following laxatives would be the most effective in lowering his serum ammonia levels?

   a. Docusate sodium (Colace).
   b. Polyethylene glyco-electrolyle solution (GoLYTELY).

   c. Lactulose (Chronulac).
   d. Sorbitol.

10. After surgery for a peptic ulcer, Mr. J. is receiving morphine sulfate 2 mg q4h, tetracycline 250 mg q6h, cimetidine (Tagamet) 300 mg q6h, and acetaminophen (Tylenol) 600 mg q4h. Which of the medications above is most likely to cause constipation?

    a. Tetracycline.
    b. Cimetidine (Tagamet).

    c. Morphine sulfate.
    d. Acetaminophen (Tylenol).

## Critical thinking case study

Mrs. J. is having diarrhea as a result of a continuous tube feeding and antibiotic therapy that she is receiving. Her physician orders a psyllium preparation (Metamucil).

1. Identify what you will do.

Mrs. J. is taken off the tube feeding and started on a regular diet. After two days on regular food, she has not had a bowel movement.

2. Discuss how you will proceed.

Two days later, Mrs. J. still has not had a bowel movement. You contact the physician and he asks you what you think would work best for Mrs. J.

3. Identify your response and your rationale for your response.

# CHAPTER 65

# Antidiarrheals

## True or false

_____ 1. Very hot foods can cause diarrhea.

_____ 2. Persons with a deficiency of lactase will have diarrhea when they eat dairy products.

_____ 3. Antibacterial agents may cause diarrhea by altering the normal bowel flora.

_____ 4. Diarrhea can be a symptom of stress in certain individuals.

_____ 5. Hypothyroidism increases bowel motility.

_____ 6. Chronic diarrhea can result in malnutrition and anemia.

_____ 7. Psyllium preparations (Metamucil) are useful for both diarrhea and constipation.

_____ 8. Withholding fluids is an effective way of treating diarrhea.

_____ 9. Intestinal tumors can cause diarrhea.

_____ 10. The drug of choice for treating diarrhea resulting from chronic inflammatory bowel disease is diphenoxylate with atropine sulfate (Lomotil).

_____ 11. Cholestyramine (Questran) is the drug of choice for treating diarrhea due to bile salts.

_____ 12. Loperamide (Imodium) is contraindicated for treating diarrhea due to bile salts.

_____ 13. Side effects of diphenoxylate (Lomotil) include bradycardia and elevated blood sugar.

_____ 14. Alcohol will decrease the effect of antidiarrheal drugs.

_____ 15. You should report to a physician if your diarrhea persists for more than 3 days.

## Review questions

1. Which of the following medications is used to treat the diarrhea associated with bacillary dysentery caused by *Shigella* organisms?
   a. Ampicillin (Omnipen).
   b. Cholestyramine (Questran).
   c. Kaolin (Donnagel).
   d. Psyllium preparations (Metamucil).

2. Sulfasalazine (Azulfidine) is most effective in treating the diarrhea associated with
   a. Crohn's disease.
   b. Malabsorption syndrome.
   c. Salmonella infection.
   d. Ulcerative colitis.

3. Which of the following medications, if administered with diphenoxylate with atropine sulfate (Lomotil), will increase their antidiarrheal effects?
   a. Narcotic analgesics.
   b. Cholinergic agents.
   c. Calcium channel blockers.
   d. Beta adrenergic blockers.

4. Which of the following statements by Mrs. B. leads you to believe that she has understood the teaching that you have done regarding diphenoxylate with atropine sulfate (Lomotil)?
   a. "It is not uncommon for there to be an increase in diarrhea initially."
   b. "I may experience dry mouth and blurred vision from this medication."
   c. "I should take the medication with foods high in vitamin C."
   d. "If I have a weight gain of more than 2 lbs. I will contact my physician."

5. The nurse should assess for which of the following adverse reactions to loperamide (Imodium)?
   a. Nausea and vomiting.
   b. Bradycardia and hypertension.
   c. Abdominal distention.
   d. A papular rash.

6. This medication is helpful in treating diarrhea secondary to malabsorption syndrome due to the deficiency of pancreatic enzymes:
   a. Pectin (Parepectolin).
   b. Lactobacillus (Bacid).
   c. Pancreatin (Viokase).
   d. Colestipol (Colestid).

7. Diphenoxylate with atropine sulfate (Lomotil) is contraindicated in
   a. persons over the age of 65.
   b. persons with diabetes.
   c. persons with renal disease.
   d. children under the age of 2.

8. Which of the following antidiarrheal medications can also be used to treat constipation?
   a. cholestyramine (Questran).
   b. Psyllium preparations (Metamucil).
   c. Loperamide (Imodium).
   d. Neomycin.

9. Mrs. J. calls you because 6-month-old J.B. has been having diarrhea for 2 days. What advice should you give her?
   a. Make sure J.B. takes in 2–3 liters of water every day.
   b. Restrict J.B.'s oral intake to decrease bowel stimulation.
   c. You need to replace fluids and electrolytes.
   d. Give J.B. dry crackers and cereal and only sips of water.

10. Which of the following instructions should you give to Mr. J. who is taking paregoric for severe diarrhea?
    a. Always take the medication on an empty stomach.
    b. Add at least 30 cc of water to each dose.
    c. Take the medication after each diarrheal stool until the diarrhea is controlled.
    d. If the medication does not control the diarrhea in 2 weeks, contact your physician.

## Critical thinking case study

You are a hospice nurse caring for Mr. N. who has a nonoperable cancerous intestinal tumor and is receiving diphenoxylate with atropine sulfate (Lomotil) to help control his diarrhea. (The learner may need to use additional sources to answer the questions below.)

1. Identify the instructions you will give Mr. N.

2. Identify the nursing assessments that you will make each visit.

Mr. N. continues to have diarrhea and is having a significant amount of abdominal pain. His physician orders 1–2 mg of morphine q2h.

3. Identify how you will proceed.

# CHAPTER 66

# Antiemetics

## Matching exercise: terms and concepts

_____ 1. A benzodiazepine useful in treating persons who experience anticipatory nausea and vomiting.

_____ 2. A corticosteroid used for treatment of nausea and vomiting.

_____ 3. An anticholinergic drug effective in treating motion sickness.

_____ 4. Administered 30 minutes before cisplatin to prevent/minimize nausea and vomiting.

_____ 5. Administered orally at 5-minute intervals until vomiting stops.

_____ 6. Used during surgical procedures to prevent nausea and vomiting.

_____ 7. These drugs block the action of acetylcholine in the brain.

_____ 8. These drugs block dopamine from receptor sites in the brain.

_____ 9. The vomiting center is located here.

_____ 10. Along with hydroxyzine (Vistaril), one of the most commonly used antiemetic agents.

A. Dexamethasone (Decadron).

B. Metoclopramide (Reglan).

C. Phosphorated carbohydrate solution (Emetrol).

D. Antihistamines.

E. Medulla oblongata.

F. Promethazine (Phenergan).

G. Phenothiazines.

H. Droperidol (Inapsine).

I. Scopolamine (Transderm Scop).

J. Lorazepam (Ativan).

K. Cerebrum.

## Review questions

1. Which of the following medications, if administered concurrently with antiemetic agents, will increase their effects?

   a. Antianxiety agents.
   b. Thiazide diuretics.
   c. Antidiarrheals.
   d. Beta adrenergic blockers.

2. The physician orders dronabinol (Marinol) for the management of Mrs. G.'s nausea and vomiting associated with her chemotherapy. Two days after starting the medication you find that Mrs. G. has a pulse rate of 58, a BP of 188/96, a macular rash, and she is anxious. Which of the following symptoms above may be related to the use of dronabinol (Marinol)?

   a. Bradycardia.
   b. Hypertension.
   c. Rash.
   d. Anxiety.

3. Persons using phenothiazines need to be assessed for extrapyramidal symptoms which include

   a. dysphoria, drowsiness, and dizziness.
   b. dyskinesia, dystonia, and akathisia.
   c. dry mouth, blurred vision, and urinary retention.
   d. hypotension, confusion, and shuffling gait.

4. Mrs. J. is to receive metoclopramide (Reglan) for nausea. Which of the following statements by Mrs. J. leads you to believe that she has understood the teaching that you have done?

    a. "During episodes of nausea, I will drink clear liquids."

    b. "I may be drowsy as a result of taking this medication."

    c. "This medication should be taken on a full stomach."

    d. "I will need to take supplemental potassium while I am taking this medication."

5. Before administering an antiemetic to a patient experiencing nausea and vomiting, the nurse should assess

    a. blood pressure.

    b. heart rate.

    c. weight.

    d. bowel sounds.

6. The use of prochlorperazine (Compazine) is contraindicated in

    a. children under the age of 12 years.

    b. preoperative patients.

    c. pregnant women.

    d. persons under 100 lbs.

7. Which of the following antiemetics is the drug of choice for use with children?

    a. Promethazine (Phenergan).

    b. Benzquinamide (Emete-Con).

    c. Buclizine (Bucladin-S).

    d. Cyclizine (Marezine).

8. Mr. P. is going on an ocean cruise and asks his physician for an antiemetic. Which of the following medications would be most effective for motion sickness?

    a. Meclizine (Antivert).

    b. Diphenhydramine (Benadryl).

    c. Hydroxyzine (Atarax).

    d. Timethobenzamide (Tigan).

9. Mr. J. has terminal cancer and has been experiencing nausea and vomiting. His physician orders a scopolamine (Transderm Scop) patch. Which statement by Mr. J. leads you to believe that he understands how to use the patch?

    a. "I will put it on in the morning and take it off at night."

    b. "I will place the patch behind my ear and replace it every 3 days."

    c. "I will place the patch on the front or back of my cheek."

    d. "I will apply a thin layer of lotion before I apply the patch to prevent irritation."

10. When administering hydroxyzine (Vistaril) to Mr. S., the nurse needs to assess Mr. S. for anticholinergic effects which include

    a. dry mouth and urinary retention.

    b. hypotension and bradycardia.

    c. dizziness and depression.

    d. drowsiness and anorexia.

## Critical thinking case study

After radiation therapy, Mrs. B., who has a 10-year history of hypertension, experiences nausea and vomiting. Her physician orders lorazepam (Ativan).

1. Discuss why this medication was ordered.

2. Identify other measures that may be helpful in controlling nausea and vomiting.

Mrs. B.'s nausea and vomiting continues, so her physician adds prochlorperazine (Compazine).

3. Explain why this drug was chosen and the expected outcome after the drug is administered.

# SECTION XI

# Drugs Used in Special Conditions

## CHAPTER 67

# Antineoplastics

## Matching exercise: terms and concepts

Match the antineoplastic agent with the disease process it is used for.

_____ 1. Chronic granulocytic leukemia.

_____ 2. Hodgkin's disease.

_____ 3. Multiple myeloma.

_____ 4. To prevent the rejection of renal transplants.

_____ 5. Acute lymphoblastic leukemia in children.

_____ 6. Carcinoma of the breast.

_____ 7. Malignant melanomas.

_____ 8. Advanced prostatic cancer.

_____ 9. Advanced endometrial carcinoma.

_____ 10. Rhabdomyosarcoma, Wilms' tumor.

_____ 11. Squamous cell carcinoma.

_____ 12. Palliation of ovarian cancer.

_____ 13. Cancer of the testes, bladder, ovaries.

_____ 14. Advanced breast cancer in postmenopausal women.

_____ 15. Used as an adjunct for palliation of symptoms in acute leukemia, Hodgkin's disease.

A. Melphalan (Alkeran).

B. Methotrexate (Mexate).

C. Medroxyprogesterone (Depo Provera).

D. Busulfan (Myleran).

E. Dactinomycin (Cosmegen).

F. Goserelin (Zoladex).

G. Semustine (Methyl-CCNU).

H. Fluorouracil (5-FU) (Adrucil).

I. Azathioprine (Imuran).

J. Cyclophosphamide (Cytoxan).

K. Carboplatin (Paraplatin).

L. Bleomycin (Blenoxane).

M. Tamoxifen (Nolvadex).

N. Prednisone (Meticorten).

O. Cisplatin (Platinol).

## True or false

_____ 1. Mitosis occurs during the S phase of cell reproduction.

_____ 2. Viruses have been linked to the development of certain types of cancers.

_____ 3. The incidence of cancer of the stomach is higher in the U.S. than in Japan.

_____ 4. Lung cancer is the leading cause of cancer death in both men and women.

_____ 5. Cancers of the mouth, throat, and esophagus are associated with excessive use of alcohol.

_____ 6. A diet high in fat has been linked to breast cancer.

_____ 7. Multiple myeloma is derived from epithelial tissue and is the most common type of malignant tumor.

_____ 8. Antineoplastic drugs that are cell-cycle specific and need to be administered continuously.

_____ 9. Alkylating agents such as nitrogen mustard act during the dividing and resting stages.

_____ 10. Alkaloids are derived from plants.

_____ 11. A blood test for carcinoembryonic antigen (CEA) is an accurate blood test commonly used for the diagnosis of cancer.

_____ 12. Alopecia is a common side effect of several antineoplastic medications.

_____ 13. The rapid breakdown or destruction of malignant cells can result in hypercalcemia.

_____ 14. If extravasation of a chemotherapeutic agent occurs, the nurse should apply warm compresses and elevate the extremity.

_____ 15. Antineoplastic drugs can exert adverse effects on nurses who prepare and administer these drugs.

## Review questions

1. An example of a cell-cycle nonspecific medication used for the treatment of cancer is
   a. asparaginase (Elspar).
   b. hydroxyurea (Hydrea).
   c. busulfan (Myleran).
   d. dacarbazine (DTIC-Dome).

2. Antimetabolites exert their cytotoxic effects only during the
   a. $G_1$ phase.
   b. S phase.
   c. $G_2$ phase.
   d. M phase.

3. Which of the following antineoplastic medications are commonly used to treat prostatic cancer?
   a. Antibiotics.
   b. Alkaloids.
   c. Hormones.
   d. Alkylating agents.

4. Mr. J. wants to know why he must have cisplatin (Platinol) weekly. He asks you why he can't have it every day and get it over with. Your best response would be:
   a. "The doctor knows what is best for you and this is the routine he has chosen."
   b. "If this medication is given daily, drug resistance will develop."
   c. "Certain drugs are more effective when given intermittently and your body also is able to rest between treatments."
   d. "If you feel that you would like to try taking the medication daily, I will contact your physician."

5. While mechlorethamine (Mustargen) is infusing intravenously, the nurse notices that it has infiltrated. What should he or she do first?
   a. Stop the infusion and administer the recommended antidote.
   b. Slow the infusion and apply ice to the area.
   c. Change the IV site and continue the infusion.
   d. Discontinue the IV, elevate the extremity, and apply heat.

6. Mr. J., who is receiving carmustine (BCNU) for Hodgkin's disease, has a low platelet count. The nurse should be observing for
   a. difficulty in breathing.
   b. bleeding.
   c. infection.
   d. confusion.

7. Mrs. P. develops stomatitis and her physician orders viscous lidocaine swish 15 minutes before meals. Identify what the nurse should be assessing for before giving Mrs. P her tray.

   a. Respiratory distress.
   b. Tachycardia.
   c. Difficulty in swallowing.
   d. Headache.

8. The nursing diagnosis that is a priority for Mrs. P., who has stomatitis secondary to the administration of chemotherapeutic agents, is

   a. impaired skin integrity.
   b. high risk for infection.
   c. alteration in nutrition.
   d. high risk for bleeding.

9. Which of the following drugs, if administered with mercaptopurine (Purinethol), will increase its effect?

   a. Allopurinol (Zyloprim).
   b. Furosemide (Lasix).
   c. Propranolol (Inderal).
   d. Verapamil (Calan).

10. When administering bleomycin (Blenoxane) to Mr. H., the nurse should assess him for

    a. tachycardia and hypertension.
    b. confusion.
    c. seizures.
    d. stomatitis and alopecia.

## Critical thinking case study

Mrs. J. is receiving doxorubicin (Adriamycin) and cyclophosphamide (Cytoxan) for breast cancer.

1. Identify what adverse effects of these drugs you will discuss with Mrs. J. and interventions that will be helpful to deal with the adverse effects.

Mrs. J. begins to lose her hair and is extremely depressed.

2. Describe how you will respond to Mrs. J.

Mrs. J. calls you to come quick because there is blood in her urine. You examine the urine and find that it is red.

3. Discuss what your nursing actions will be.

One week after the initial treatment you find that Mrs. J. has a respiratory rate of 28 and a pulse of 102 and rales are audible in her lung bases bilaterally.

4. Describe what you will do next.

# CHAPTER 68

# Drugs Used in Ophthalmic Conditions

## Matching exercise: terms and concepts

_____ 1  May follow topical steroid therapy or injury.

_____ 2.  May be caused by inadequate lacrimation.

_____ 3.  A chronic infection in the lash follicles on the eyelid.

_____ 4.  Characterized by redness and watery discharge.

_____ 5.  Increased intraocular pressure.

_____ 6.  White, opaque fibrous tissue that covers 5/6 of the eyeball.

_____ 7.  The innermost layer of the eyeball.

_____ 8.  Constriction of the pupil.

_____ 9.  Dilation of the pupil.

_____ 10.  An elastic transparent structure that focuses light rays to form images on the retina.

A. Glaucoma.

B. Conjunctivitis.

C. Blepharitis.

D. Keratitis.

E. Corneal ulcer.

F. Retina

G. Miosis.

H. Lens.

I. Mydriasis.

J. Sclera.

K. Cornea.

## Complete the following sentences

1. Acute glaucoma may be precipitated by the following drugs: _____, _____ _____, _____, and antidepressants.

2. Corticosteroids such as dexamethasone (Decadron Phosphate) are used to treat _____ of the eye.

3. A carbonic anhydrase inhibitor such as acetazolamide (Diamox) _____ intraocular pressure.

4. Fluorescein is a _____ used to diagnose lesions or foreign bodies in the eye.

5. A cholinergic drug _____ is instilled in the eye _____ times per day and causes the pupil to _____.

6. Anticholinergic drugs such as atropine are used prior to eye exams to _____ the pupil; their use is usually contraindicated in the presence of _____.

7. To administer eye drops, have the client look _____, then pull the _____ and drop the medication in the _____.

8. The person receiving eye medications should be aware that local effects include: _____, _____, _____, _____, and allergic conjunctivitis.

9. Long-term use of anticholinesterase agents such as physostigmine salicylate (Isopto Eserine) may cause _____.

10. When miotic drugs such as pilocarpine are administered, the client may experience

_____.

## Name that drug

Identify the medications that cause the following adverse effects:

1. Dehydration and hyperglycemia. _____

2. Bradycardia and bronchoconstriction. _____

3. Dry mouth and tachycardia. _____

4. Nausea and paresthesias. _____

5. Hypertension and arrhythmias. _____

## Drug classifications

Give an example of one drug in each classification and what it is used for.

|  | **Medication** | **Use** |
| --- | --- | --- |
| 1. Adrenergic | | |
| 2. Antiadrenergic | | |
| 3. Cholinergic | | |
| 4. Anticholinesterase | | |
| 5. Anticholinergic | | |
| 6. Carbonic anhydrase inhibitor | | |
| 7. Osmotic agents | | |
| 8. Anesthetics | | |
| 9. Antiallergic | | |
| 10. Antiseptic | | |

## Review questions

1. When administering an ophthalmic medication, you should pull the
   a. lower lid down and drop the medication in the conjunctival sac.
   b. lower lid down and drop the medication on the eye, being careful not to touch it with the applicator.
   c. upper lid up and have the person look down.
   d. upper lid up and place the medication in the center of the eye.

2. Your client with glaucoma is to go home on dipivefrin (Propine) 1 gtt. q12h. Your instructions should include the following information:
   a. "When administering eye medications, you may experience redness, discomfort, and tearing."
   b. "Nausea, vomiting, and diarrhea are common side effects of all ophthalmic medications."
   c. "Lie down for 5 minutes after taking the medications."
   d. "If you experience headaches, decrease the dose to once a day."

3. Pilocarpine, a cholinergic miotic, reduces intraocular pressure by
   a. contracting the sphincter muscle of the eye.
   b. preventing ciliary muscle spasm.
   c. decreasing production of aqueous humor.
   d. increasing outflow of aqueous humor.

4. Clients receiving pilocarpine (Pilocar) will experience
   a. miosis.
   b. mydriasis.
   c. no pupillary change.
   d. double vision.

5. Side effects that a person receiving carbonic anhydrase inhibitors such as Diamox might experience include
   a. dehydration and hyperglycemia.
   b. bradycardia and bronchoconstriction.
   c. nausea and paresthesias.
   d. hypertension and dysrhythmias.

6. Which of the following statements demonstrates that the client understands the teaching you have done about pilocarpine?
   a. "I know I must eat food high in potassium and stay away from salt."
   b. "I know that I will have decreased vision in dim light so I don't plan to drive at night."
   c. "The dosage of pilocarpine will need to be increased as I get older."
   d. "I can no longer operate heavy machinery."

7. Lubricants are used for
   a. conjunctivitis.
   b. blepharitis.
   c. keratitis.
   d. corneal ulcers.

8. A dye used to diagnose lesions or foreign bodies in the eye is
   a. atropine.
   b. mannitol.
   c. dexamethasone.
   d. fluorescein.

9. Which of the following agents is used in newborns to prevent eye damage from gonorrhea?
   a. Cromolyn sodium.
   b. Mannitol.
   c. Silver nitrate.
   d. Gentamicin.

10. Your client has glaucoma. Which of these medications ordered preoperatively should be questioned because it can precipitate acute glaucoma?
   a. Atropine.
   b. Demerol.
   c. Vistaril.
   d. Gentamicin.

## Critical thinking case study

Mrs. R. has come to the office for an eye exam because she had difficulty in threading a needle. Her intraocular pressure is significantly elevated so her physician orders timolol maleate (Timoptic) and pilocarpine (Pilocar).

1.  Discuss why these medications were ordered for Mrs. R.

2.  Identify the instructions that you will give Mrs. R.

Mrs. R. complains of burning when she instills the drops and asks you how long she will have to continue taking these drops.

3.  Discuss how you will respond to Mrs. R.

Mrs. R.'s brother also has glaucoma and she is concerned about her children.

4.  Discuss how you will respond to Mrs. R.

# CHAPTER 69

# Drugs Used in Dermatologic Conditions

## Matching exercise: terms and concepts

_____ 1. Pigment-producing cells.

_____ 2. An inflammatory response of the skin to various injuries.

_____ 3. "Hives."

_____ 4. Chronic skin disorder characterized by dry scaling lesions.

_____ 5. Characterized by erythema, tenderness, and edema.

_____ 6. An infection of the hair follicles.

_____ 7. "Boils."

_____ 8. A contagious skin infection.

_____ 9. This fungal infection can occur following the use of broad-spectrum antibiotics.

_____ 10. "Athlete's foot."

_____ 11. A viral infection of the skin.

_____ 12. Follicles become infected, and pustules, cysts, and abscesses are formed.

_____ 13. A drying agent used for exudative lesions.

_____ 14. An agent used to debride wounds.

_____ 15. An agent used to remove warts.

_____ 16. An oil-based substance useful in chronic skin conditions characterized by dry lesions.

_____ 17. These substances may be used on the face or hairy, moist areas.

_____ 18. Suspensions of insoluble substances that cool, dry, and protect the skin.

_____ 19. A substance that absorbs, cools, and protects.

_____ 20. A semi-solid preparation that adheres strongly to the area of application.

A. Dermatitis.

B. Psoriasis.

C. Folliculitis.

D. Impetigo.

E. Tinea pedis.

F. Warts.

G. Astringent.

H. Enzyme.

I. Acne vulgaris.

J. Oral candidiasis.

K. Furuncles.

L. Cellulitis.

M. Urticaria.

N. Melanocytes.

O. Keratolytic agent.

P. Creams.

Q. Powders.

R. Paste.

S. Lotion.

T. Ointment.

## Review questions

1. Mrs. J. states that she applies Neosporin Ointment to every cut that her son gets. Identify the best reply to Mrs. J.'s statement.

    a. Lesions can occur with chronic use of Neosporin.

    b. That is an excellent idea; it will prevent your son from developing an infection.

    c. Drug resistance can develop with overuse of topical antibiotics.

    d. When the skin is broken, more of the drug is absorbed systemically, so you need to observe for toxic side effects of the medication.

2. One of the most effective topical agents for acne is

    a. Neosporin.

    b. benzoyl peroxide.

    c. chlorhexidine (Hibiclens).

    d. pHisohex.

3. Mrs. P. is applying cornstarch to J.J.'s perineal area every time she changes his diaper. What instructions will you give her?

    a. Cornstarch may promote growth of bacteria and fungi.

    b. Cornstarch is very drying to the skin; only use it when J.J. has a rash.

    c. Cornstarch should be applied no more than four times a day.

    d. Apply the cornstarch on J.J.'s diaper, not directly to his skin.

4. The physician orders tretinoin (Retin-A) for Miss H.'s acne. Which of the following instructions should the nurse give to Miss H.?

    a. You should see positive results from the medication within 1 week.

    b. Wash your face before each application and use it in the morning and at bedtime.

    c. You should leave the medication on for an hour, then remove it with soap and water.

    d. Apply the medication no more than once a day. Overuse will cause severe inflammation.

5. Miss P. is using isotretinoin (Accutane) for severe acne. Which of the following statements by Miss P. leads you to believe that she has understood the teaching that you have done?

    a. "I will increase my intake of foods high in vitamin K."

    b. "I will avoid extended exposure to direct sunlight."

    c. "I will wash my face four times a day and apply the medication after each washing."

    d. "After 4-6 weeks of using this drug, my acne should clear up."

6. B.H. has a rash in his axillae. His physician prescribes amcinonide (Cyclocort). An adverse effect of excessive administration of topical steroids is

    a. atrophy of the skin.

    b. superinfection.

    c. cracking and splitting of the skin.

    d. loss of pigmentation in the area of application.

7. Identify which of the following agents is the drug of choice for treating psoriasis:

    a. Resorcinol.

    b. Acetic acid.

    c. Gentian violet.

    d. Sulfur.

8. P.G. has been exposed to poison ivy. Which of the following medications would be most helpful to relieve her itching?

    a. Coal tar (Balnetar).

    b. Colloidal oatmeal (Aveeno).

    c. Trioxsalen (Trisoralen).

    d. Sutilains (Travase).

9. Mr. J. is being treated with isotretinoin (Accutane) for severe acne. The nurse should be assessing Mr. J. for which of the following adverse responses to the medication?

   a. Nausea, vomiting, and blurred vision.    c. Hair loss.

   b. Hypertension and arrhythmias.    d. Anorexia and diarrhea.

10. Mr. R. is started on haloprogin (Halotex) for tinea pedis (athlete's feet). Which of the following statements by Mr. R. leads you to believe that he has understood the teaching that you have done regarding Halotex?

    a. "I will apply the ointment daily for 6 weeks."    c. "I will soak my feet in cold water before each application."

    b. "I will use the powder three times a day and only wear white socks for the next month."    d. "I will apply the medication at morning and bedtime for 2–4 weeks."

## Critical thinking case study

M., a 19-year-old college student, comes to the clinic to be treated for acne. She was previously treated at age 16 with tetracycline with limited success. The physician starts her on tretinoin (Retin-A).

1. Identify what instructions you will give M.

M. returns 1 month later. Her face acne is worse. She states that she has started taking birth control pills.

2. Identify the teaching that you will do with M.

Two months after she has received the medication, M. returns. Her face is excoriated. She admits to using the tretinoin (Retin-A) four times a day.

3. Identify what you will do.

# CHAPTER 70

# Drug Use During Pregnancy and Lactation

## Drug interactions

Place an X next to the drugs that should be avoided during pregnancy.

_____ 1. Captopril (Capoten).

_____ 2. Thiazide diuretics.

_____ 3. Penicillins.

_____ 4. Aminoglycosides.

_____ 5. Tetracyclines.

_____ 6. Corticosteroids.

_____ 7. Laxatives.

_____ 8. Oral antidiabetic agents.

_____ 9. Quinidine (Quinaglute).

_____ 10. Antimanic agent.

_____ 11. Alcohol.

_____ 12. Nicotine (cigarette smoking).

## Matching exercise: terms and concepts

_____ 1. Stimulate uterine contraction; used to initiate the birth process.

_____ 2. Cause relaxation of uterine smooth muscle.

_____ 3. Used to stimulate labor when uterine contractions are weak and ineffective.

_____ 4. The drug of choice for treating pain during labor.

_____ 5. Used after delivery of the baby if bleeding is severe.

_____ 6. Used to suppress lactation.

A. Ritodrine (Yutopar).

B. Meperidine (Demerol).

C. Ergonovine maleate (Ergotrate).

D. Bromocriptine (Parlodel).

E. Oxytocin (Pitocin).

F. Prostaglandins.

G. Morphine.

## Complete the following sentences

### NORMAL PREGNANCY

#### Vascular System

1. Cardiac output _____ 30–40% above nonpregnant level at approximately 24th week of gestation.

2. ____% _____ in circulating blood volume because of an _____ in plasma renin levels stimulate the secretion of aldosterone causing retention of NA+ and $H_2O$.

3. Physiologic _____ develops because of hemodilution of the blood volume.

4. Decreased peripheral resistance. There is dilation of the arterial system causing pooling of blood. Therefore, BP does not go up even though there is a substantial _____ in blood volume.

### PREGNANCY-INDUCED HYPERTENSION

1. Hypovolemia despite fluid retention because the fluid shifts into the interstitial space causing _____.

2. Decreased platelet count, chronic intravascular coagulation leading to hemolytic _____.

3. Increased peripheral resistance and vasoconstriction which leads to increased ____.

#### Renal System

5. _____ glomerular filtration rate (GFR) up to 50% increase to clear creatinine, urea, and uric acid more quickly.

4. _____ glomerular filtration rate; therefore, increased levels of uric acid (which are associated with poor fetal outcome).

5. _____ protein loss, _____ NA+ and $H_2O$, _____ urinary output.

#### Gastrointestinal System

6. _____ peristalsis.
7. _____ abdominal pressure.

## Crossword puzzle

### Across

1. Many drugs given to the mother can be transmitted to neonates via ____.
3. Analgesic of choice for use during labor.
4. Drugs administered to the mother particularly affect this fetal organ.
7. A lactation-suppressant drug.
8. Used during pregnancy for chronic hypertension.
9. For diabetic women, _____ requirements vary throughout pregnancy.
10. Possible side effects of this drug include hypotension and water intoxication.

### Down

2. Preferred analgesic for minor aches and pains during pregnancy.
5. A type of drug given to inhibit labor contractions.
6. Administered to the mother for its therapeutic effect on fetal tachycardia.

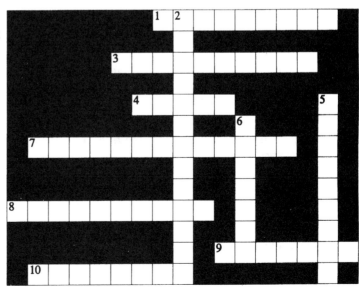

## Review questions

1. Which of the following drugs is known to be excreted in breast milk and not recommended for use by nursing mothers?
   a. Hydrochlorothiazide (Hydrodiuril).
   b. Digoxin (Lanoxin).
   c. Heparin.
   d. Diphenoxylate (Lomotil).

2. Mrs. J. comes to the hospital in labor. She is 6 months pregnant and her physician tries to stop her labor with ritodrine (Yutopar). Which of the following assessments will you do on an ongoing basis?
   a. Fetal heart rate.
   b. Hourly urinary outputs.
   c. Deep tendon reflexes.
   d. Level of consciousness.

3. Water intoxication and seizures are adverse effects associated with the administration of large doses of
   a. ritodrine (Yutopar).
   b. oxytocin (Pitocin).
   c. meperidine (Demerol).
   d. terbutaline (Brethine).

4. Mrs. G. is receiving magnesium sulfate because her blood pressure was 168/90 before her labor started. An indication of toxicity caused by magnesium sulfate that the nurse should be assessing for is
   a. an apical pulse below 60.
   b. a respiratory rate above 28.
   c. an increased blood pressure.
   d. absent deep tendon reflexes.

5. The physician orders 2 g of magnesium sulfate in 100 ml of 5 DW to infuse over 15 minutes. The IMED delivers ml/hr. How will you set the IMED to deliver the correct amount of medication?
   a. 100 ml/hr.
   b. 200 ml/hr.
   c. 300 ml/hr.
   d. 400 ml/hr.

6. After Mrs. H. delivers, she is given ergonovine maleate (Ergotrate). The purpose of this drug is to
   a. suppress lactation.
   b. stimulate lactation.
   c. suppress uterine bleeding.
   d. suppress uterine contraction.

7. Mrs. P. receives bromocriptine (Parlodel) for suppression of lactation. What other instructions would be helpful to prevent breast engorgement?
   a. Drink plenty of fluids.
   b. Wear a bra that gives you good support.
   c. Take warm showers and massage your breasts if you feel tender.
   d. Expressing the milk will help you feel more comfortable.

8. A drug commonly used to treat hypertension in pregnant women is
   a. hydrochorothiazide (Hydrodiuril).
   b. minoxidil (Loniten).
   c. methyldopa (Adomet).
   d. captopril (Capoten).

9. Mrs. J. has been on oral antidiabetic agents for 3 years. When she becomes pregnant, the doctor decides to put her on insulin. Mrs. J. asks you, "Why do I have to be on insulin?" The best response would be:
   a. The doctor knows what is best for you. He is doing this to try and maintain your pregnancy.
   b. Your insulin requirements will vary throughout your pregnancy and insulin can be adjusted as needed.
   c. You need to discuss this with your doctor; maybe he can control your diabetes with diet.
   d. Oral agents cause hypoglycemia in the fetus and insulin does not.

10. Mrs. G. is 8 months pregnant and complaining of constipation. Which of the following instructions will you give her?
    a. You can use docusate sodium (Colace) three times a day until your constipation improves.
    b. Bulk-producing laxatives are the safest for the fetus.
    c. Mineral oil is very effective. Take it at bedtime.
    d. Take 2 Senokot followed by hot liquids every 2 hours until you have a bowel movement.

## Critical thinking case study

Mrs. J. is brought to the hospital. She has been leaking amniotic fluid for 2 days and her physician has decided to induce her. He orders a prostaglandin vaginal suppository, to be followed by an oxytocin (Pitocin) drip. Mrs. J. is extremely apprehensive and asks you why she must receive these medications.

1. Describe how you will respond to Mrs. J.

Two hours after the initiation of the oxytocin drip, Mrs. J. complains of severe pain.

2. Identify what your nursing actions will be.

The physician orders meperidine (Demerol) IV push. Mrs. J. states that everything is going black and she appears to faint.

3. Identify and prioritize your nursing actions.

# Answers

# Answers

## CHAPTER 1
### Introduction to Pharmacology

**Matching exercises: terms and concepts**

1. D.
2. E.
3. A.
4. G.
5. B.
6. K.
7. I.
8. F.
9. H.
10. C.
11. J.
12. O.
13. L.
14. M.
15. N.

**True or false**

1. T.
2. F.
3. T.
4. T.
5. F.
6. T.
7. T.
8. T.
9. F.
10. T.
11. F.
12. T.
13. F.
14. T.
15. T.

**Cell Physiology**

*Part A*

1. Cell membrane.
2. Cytoplasm.
3. Lysosomes.
4. Nucleus.
5. Chromatin.
6. Endoplasmic reticulum.
7. Ribosomes.
8. Golgi apparatus.
9. Mitochondria.

*Part B*

Drug movement and therefore drug
  action are affected by a drug's ability
  to cross cell membranes.

**Review questions**

1. c.
2. d.
3. c.
4. a.
5. b.

6. c.
7. a.
8. b.
9. c.
10. c.

## CHAPTER 2
### Administering Medications

**Matching exercise: terms and concepts**

1. B.
2. F.
3. A.
4. C.
5. D.
6. E.
7. G.
8. H.
9. I.
10. J.
11. L.
12. O.
13. M.
14. N.
15. P.

**Abbreviations and equivalents**

*Part I. Abbreviations*

1. I.
2. F.
3. G.
4. C.
5. J.
6. K.
7. B.
8. D.
9. H.
10. A.

*Part II. Equivalents*

1. E.
2. C.
3. H.
4. K.
5. A.
6. D.
7. B.
8. F.
9. G.
10. L.

**Practice Set I**

1. 1 tablet.
2. 0.5 ml.
3. 30 ml.
4. 2 tablets.
5. 1.5 cc.
6. 0.6 cc.
7. 1.55 ml or 1.6.
8. Give 10 cc.

9. Give 3 ml.
10. Give 1 cc.
11. 5 cc.
12. 1.5 ml.

**Practice Set II**

1. 60 ml.
2. 3 tablets.
3. 360 ml.
4. 60 kilograms.
5. 1250 milliliters.
6. 2.5 ml.
7. 1.2 gms.
8. 0.4 ml.
9. 0.25 ml.
10. 2 tsp.

**Review questions**

1. d.
2. b.
3. d.
4. b.
5. c.
6. a.
7. c.
8. b.
9. b.
10. d.

## CHAPTER 3
### Nursing Process in Drug Therapy

**True or false**

1. T.
2. F.
3. T.
4. T.
5. T.
6. F.
7. T.
8. T.
9. F.
10. T.
11. T
12. F
13. T
14. T
15. T

**Review questions**

1. c.
2. d.
3. b.
4. b.
5. b.
6. a.
7. a.
8. b.
9. b.
10. a.

## CHAPTER 4
### Physiology of the Central Nervous System

#### Complete the following sentences

1. brain; spinal cord.
2. synapse; neurons.
3. acetylcholine, catecholamines, (nor-epinephrine), histamine, serotonin, endorphins, enkephalins.
4. conscious processes.
5. heat, cold, pain, muscle position sense.
6. body temperature, arterial blood pressure, anterior pituitary hor-mones, food and water intake.
7. cardiac, respiratory, vasomotor.
8. wakefulness and alertness.
9. behavior, emotions.
10. muscular activity. maintain balance, posture.
11. skeletal muscle.
12. medullary, pyramids.
13. hypoxia.
14. confusion, dizziness, convulsions, loss of consciousness, brain damage.
15. Thiamine.
16. myelin sheath; Wernicke-Korsakoff's.
17. drowsiness, decreased muscle tone, decreased ability to move, decreased perception of sensation.
18. unconsciousness, respiratory failure.
19. wakefulness, alertness, decreased fatigue.
20. hyperactivity, excessive talking, nervousness, insomnia.
21. seizures, dysrhythmias, death.

#### Neurotransmission in the central nervous system

*Part A*

1. Synapse
2. Release site.
3. Postsynaptic nerve terminal.
4. Receptor sites.
5. Postsynaptic nerve cell membrane.
6. Presynaptic nerve cell membrane.
7. Neurotransmitters.
8. Presynaptic nerve terminal.

*Part B*

1. synapse; receptor sites.
2. the postsynaptic membranes of nerve cells supplying those organs.

#### Review questions

1. a.
2. c.
3. b.
4. d.
5. b.
6. a.
7. d.
8. c.
9. a.
10. c.

## CHAPTER 5
### Narcotic Analgesics and Narcotic Antagonists

#### Complete the following sentences

1. a. drowsiness, unconsciousness.
   b. decreased mental and physical activity.
   c. respiratory depression.
   d. nausea and vomiting.
   e. pupil constriction.
2. slowing motility; constipation.
3. PO, IM, IV.
4. 20 mg, 30 mg.
5. ASA or Tylenol.
6. short acting; less respiratory depres-sion. 50–100 mg, 2–4.
7. Stadol, Nubain, Talwin.
8. Narcan.
9. assess the patient's pain.
10. a. ambulation.
    b. heat or cold.
    c. relaxation.
11. Pain threshold, placebo response, behavioral response.
12. IV; it is faster acting.
13. PCA pump.
14. 24 to 48 hrs.
15. Atropine.
16. crying, thrashing, muscle rigidity.
17. respiratory.
18. smoke; ambulate.
19. respiratory depression, hypotension, sedation, vomiting.
20. alcohol.

#### Word scramble

1. FENTANYL
2. CODEINE
3. DEMEROL
4. DILAUDID
5. MORPHINE
6. STADOL
7. DARVON
8. NUBAIN
9. NARCAN
10. TALWIN

#### Review questions

1. c.
2. b.
3. a.
4. d.
5. b.
6. a.
7. a.
8. c.
9. c.
10. b.

## CHAPTER 6
### Analgesic–Antipyretic–Anti-inflam-matory and Related Drugs

#### Matching exercise: terms and concepts

1. D.
2. E.
3. A.
4. I.
5. H.

### Chapter 5 Word Scramble

```
N O T H S B H Y P O F T I L C L C E F G H H J N K
K A D R E N E R G I C E N B E T A Z O L O L A N E
C M R I A S S A N L L X Q K E Z S V C D N C A T V
X Y Z T I P L D N E D R O N O N I R L A R N V R R
H L P O D I L A U D I D I C A Y Y O D A V V P P J
F N V A N L I C B R E E K X F H T G N A E S O S B
R I L U A A C A I D D U K L O E E U E T O R R P
X T O S H R F R N O H A Z Y P X D K B B L K A O T
L R N A Y J R E C L N O S T Y H P E A N B E R E C
V A S G O N I Q P F E N T A N Y L K I S N L O K C
X T K X T G A A N G N P A P E C O R N I U O U S A
K J K X C Z A B T N T A D P V C D T E G F G X H O
V A S D I P I O C P R A O Z O I N J K A J K L D N
O N A E S O R P T I O N L W N C I N U C N C I V O
P T O M I I A N G I N Y B W I X K U N L S I N E T
A Z A E Y B I D L E S X F N I N S V D F H I A N I
R S C R F X Z Y N G R H V T G N J N A A E Z H T L
G E M O R P H I N E V K O N M H C H L O R Z I D E
Y N O L G D B P Q E R R O T V S P Q Y L O V B P C
L W I E F I C D L S N E V H O W G Y O Z A J O W D
F D O M R G G L I I S T P R O T E R E N E R Z N X
N C O E U M A D I N S F T P T M I G J F U W T C Y
E F D D Q C N Q N T A T D Y M N S J Z E B G O G C
```

6. B.
7. G.
8. C.
9. F.
10. L.

**True or false**

1. T.
2. F.
3. F.
4. T.
5. T.

**Review questions**

1. c.
2. a.
3. a.
4. a.
5. a.
6. d.
7. c.
8. c.
9. b.
10. a.

## CHAPTER 7
### Sedative-Hypnotics

**Complete the following sentences**

1. (rapid eye movement); mentally and emotionally restorative.
2. pain, anxiety, illness, changes in lifestyle, drugs.
3. rebound effect.
4. drug-metabolizing enzymes.
5. 2 wks.
6. severe respiratory disorders, hypersensitivity reaction, alcohol or drug abuse, disease, kidney disorders.
7. tapered and gradually discontinued.
8. REM sleep, 2 wks.
9. excessive sedation, respiratory depression, shock, chronic intoxication, withdrawal or abstinence syndrome.

**True or false**

1. T.
2. T.
3. F.
4. F.
5. F.
6. F.
7. T

**Review questions**

1. b.
2. b.
3. a.
4. d.
5. d.
6. c.
7. c.
8. d.
9. b.
10. a.

## CHAPTER 8
### Antianxiety Drugs

**Complete the following sentences**

1. severe or prolonged.
2. phobias, panic, obsessive-compulsive, post-traumatic stress, atypical anxiety disorders, generalized anxiety.
3. motor tension, overactivity of the autonomic nervous system, increased vigilance.
4. benzodiazepines.
5. physical, psychological.
6. fat; plasma, proteins.
7. (Librium), (Valium), (Tranxene); long; 5–7.
8. antianxiety, hypnotic, anticonvulsant; sedation; agitation, delirium tremens.
9. severe respiratory disorders, severe liver disease, hypersensitivity reactions, history of drug abuse.
10. (BuSpar); sedation; physical; psychological; muscle relaxant; anticonvulsant.
11. (Vistaril); potentiates.
12. antiemetic, antihistamine.
13. drug tolerance, drug dependence, abuse, withdrawal symptoms.
14. 3–4.
15. increased anxiety, insomnia, irritability, headaches, tremor, palpitations. confusion, abnormal perception of movement, depersonalization, psychosis and seizures.
16. oxazepam (Serax), lorazepam (Ativan).
17. 5 mg/ml/min., large, resuscitation equipment.
18. alcohol; barbiturates, narcotic analgesics, phenothiazines, cimetidine, disulfiram, isoniazid.
19. ephedrine, pseudoephedrine, phenylpropanolamine, theophylline.

**Nursing diagnosis**

*Nursing Diagnoses*

1. Sleep pattern disturbance: insomnia.
2. Ineffective individual coping.
3. Knowledge deficit related to the appropriate use of antianxiety medications.

*Assessment*

1. Observe for physiological manifestations of anxiety, increased BP, increased pulse, increased respiratory rate, increased muscle tension.
2. a. Assess for level of anxiety.
   b. Assess effects of anxiety on: person's perception, ability to learn, problem solving.
   c. Assess coping and defense mechanism.
3. Assess for a therapeutic response to antianxiety medications.

*Nursing Interventions*

1. a. Reduce environmental stimuli.
   b. Use measures to increase comfort.
   c. Administer antianxiety medications.
2. a. Remain calm.
   b. Assist client to identify stressors.
   c. Provide outlets for excess energy.

d. Identify previous coping mechanisms.
3. a. Instruct client to avoid alcohol while taking antianxiety medications.
   b. Instruct client that antianxiety drugs are for short-term use.
   c. Ask your client pertinent questions to assess his or her knowledge regarding the medications.

*DEFINE:*

ANXIETY: a response to a stressful situation resulting in fear, apprehension, nervousness, or worry.

**Review questions**

1. d.
2. d.
3. a.
4. d.
5. a.
6. b.
7. d.
8. c.
9. c.
10. a.

## CHAPTER 9
### Antipsychotic Drugs

**Complete the following sentences**

1. Schizophrenia.
2. phenothiazines.
3. CNS depression, autonomic nervous system depression, antiemetic effect, lowering of body temperature, hypersensitivity reactions.
4. dopamine.
5. anxiety, agitation, hyperactivity, insomnia, aggressive/combative behavior, hallucinations.
6. nausea, vomiting.
7. a. ci.
   b. ci.
   c. ci.
   d. ca.
   e. ca.
   f. ci.
   g. ca.
   h. ca.
   i. ci.
   j. ci.
   k. ca.
   l. ci.
   m. ci.
8. (Taractan), (Navane); antipsychotic.
9. (Haldol); high; hypotension; sedation; high; extrapyramidal effects.
10. mental retardation with hyperkinesia, Tourette's syndrome, Huntington's disease.
11. (Loxitane); (Clozaril); agranulocytosis, sedation, orthostatic hypotension.
12. Tourette's syndrome. tardive dyskinesia, major motor seizures, sudden death.
13. alleviate symptoms, increase the client's ability to cope, promote optimal functioning.
14. respond to another; equivalent.
15. injections; fluphenazine (Prolixin).
16. once; 1–2 hrs. of.
17. 60 ml; fruit juice or water.

18. hypotension, tachycardia, dizziness, faintness, fatigue.
19. dry mouth, caries, blurred vision, constipation, paralytic ileus, urinary retention.
20. menstrual irregularities, decreased libido, weight gain; possible impotence.

### Word scramble

1. TINDAL
2. MELLARIL
3. COMPAZINE
4. PROLIXIN
5. THORAZINE
6. TRILAFON
7. SPARINE
8. STELAZINE
9. MOBAN
10. ORAP
11. CLOZARIL
12. HALDOL
13. TARACTAN
14. NAVANE
15. LOXITANE

### Review questions

1. c.
2. a.
3. d.
4. a.
5. b.
6. d.
7. b.
8. a.
9. d.
10. a.

### CHAPTER 10
### Antidepressants

#### Complete the following sentences

1. a. fatigue.
   b. indecisiveness.
   c. difficulty concentrating.
   d. loss of interest in appearance, work, sex.
   e. feelings of guilt.
   f. change in appetite.
   g. sleep disorder.
   h. somatic symptoms.
   i. obsession with death.
2. environmental stress, adverse life events, concurrent disease states.
3. sedation, orthostatic hypotension.
4. (Prozac), nausea, nervousness, insomnia, skin rash.
5. foods, drugs; hypertensive crisis.
6. tyramine.
7. a. cheese.
   b. alcohol.
   c. bananas.
   d. caffeine.
   e. chocolate.
   f. raisins.
   g. sour cream.
   h. yogurt.
8. (Eskalith), bipolar affective disorder.
9. Adequate kidney function.
10. sodium.
11. several months.
12. a lifetime.
13. 2–3 wks.
14. 0.8–1.2.
15. type, severity.
16. dry mouth, constipation, blurred vision, tachycardia, orthostatic hypertension, drowsiness, dizziness, excessive.
17. severe nausea, vomiting, diarrhea, ataxia, incoordination, dizziness, slurred speech, blurred vision, tinnitus, muscle twitching, tremors, increased muscle tone.

#### Sentence correction

1. urinary retention.
2. meperidine (Demerol); adrenergic agents, alcohol, guanethidine, levadopa, and reserpine.
3. sodium.
4. daily.
5. severe headaches.
6. renal.
7. norepinephrine.
8. arrhythmias.
9. hemodialysis.
10. nicotine.
11. 4.
12. mania.
13. physostigmine (Antilirium).
14. 2.
15. 12; 6.

#### Review questions

1. c.
2. a.
3. c.
4. d.
5. d.
6. a.
7. c.
8. a.
9. c.
10. b.

### Chapter 9 Word Scramble

```
T A L E F D F D Q C N Q N S P A R I N E T X A T W
A N C O E K N U M O A R D I Q N B P N T P T M I H
R G P T M T M I G J F U W T C Y I D E O M R G K
A G G L I I S T M N P K R O T E Z R E N R E Z N X
C L L W I N E F I C D E L S N A X U O W Y O Z A R
T Y O N R D G S D B P W B R P R O T V S P Q V Y L
A V G E M A A O R H P H I M E V K O F N M H T M I
N Z R B T L C L O I X M O B A N I X E U Z Y R N G
R H V T G H F J J N A C L O Z A R I L E A Z I H O
A T L Y A Z O Y B I D L E S P X T F N D N S L S V
D F H I M D F R U T P T O R T I D S H L B Z A T E
X O N A B Q S O A R P P T I U O N D C O W N F C I
R U C N K I V O V Z A S H Q O I P C P X R A O L Z
F K J K Z X C Z A M I B T A N D A O A I P V N C D
G C D T X E C F J G E N F G L X H O L T E B T M O
C D T I P B Q T U D H L E R A D P D A A P X D A T
P L A A W S M A X V T G L A A G O N P N A P E C N
O R R N I U O Q U S P U S A V A S L G E O N E I Q
P O F E J N T N A N Y L K I R S B N C L K I S N L
O K C P L V R N A I A Y J R E I C L N O S W T Y H
P E A R B S E R E V C X T S T E L A Z I N E T O S
P R O L I X I N X A A S O N I Q U G P E N T A N Y
L K I S N G L O O K L N R N A Y J R E C L I N O S
T Y H P E A M B E R E C E P X T O S H R F R N O H
H M A Z Y P X D R M B B L K A O T R I L U A A C B
```

## CHAPTER 11
### Anticonvulsants

#### Complete the following sentences

1. Brief episode of abnormal electrical activity.
2. type of seizure characterized by spasmodic contractions of involuntary muscles.
3. chronic recurrent pattern of seizures.
4. EEG.
5. developmental defects, metabolic disease, birth injury.
6. children; phenytoin.
7. 10–20 µg.
8. (Valium; acute convulsive seizures.
9. Carbamazepine, cannot be controlled by other drugs. trigeminal neuralgia.
10. brain surgery, head injury, drug overdose.
11. life-long.
12. weeks or months.
13. normal saline, precipitate.
14. hypotension, dysrhythmias, depression, cardiac arrest.
15. folic acid.

#### True or false

1. T.
2. F.
3. F.
4. T.
5. F.
6. F.
7. T.

#### Crossword puzzle

*Across*

2. Klonopin
4. Tranxene
5. Valium
9. Phenobarbital

*Down*

1. Convulsion
3. Tegretol
6. Dilantin
7. Depakene
8. Epilepsy
10. Ativan

#### Review questions

1. a.
2. c.
3. b.

4. a.
5. b.
6. d.
7. c.
8. a.
9. d.
10. d.

## CHAPTER 12
### Anti-Parkinson Drugs

#### Complete the following sentences

1. chronic, progressive, degenerative; tremor, bradykinesia, joint and muscle rigidity.
2. dopamine; acetylcholine.
3. levodopa, (Lodosyn) (Symmetrel), (Parlodel).
4. (Symmetrel); dopamine release.
5. (Parlodel); postsynaptic dopamine receptors.
6. glaucoma, gastrointestinal obstruction, prostate hypertrophy, urinary bladder, neck obstruction, myasthenia gravis.
7. most effective.
8. recurrence.
9. (Sinemet); brain.
10. (Symmetrel); 1–5.
11. (Parlodel); prolong the effectiveness; required dose.
12. bradykinesia and rigidity.

#### True or false

1. F.
2. T.
3. T.
4. F.
5. F.
6. F.

#### Review questions

1. d.
2. c.
3. d.
4. a.
5. b.
6. a.
7. b.
8. d.
9. a.
10. c.

## CHAPTER 13
### Skeletal Muscle Relaxants

#### Complete the following sentences

1. decrease muscle spasms; spasticity.
2. Dantrolene (Dantrium).
3. hyperthermia.
4. mental alertness; physical coordination.
5. baclofen (Lioresal).
6. diazepam (Valium), methocarbamol (Robaxin), orphenadrine citrate (Norflex).
7. a. massage, moist heat, and exercise.
   b. bedrest for acute muscle spasm.
   c. relaxation techniques.
   d. correct posture and lifting.
8. children under 12.
9. 2 mg/min., respiratory depression and apnea.
10. (Soma), bradycardia, hypotension, dizziness.

#### True or false

1. T.
2. F.
3. F.
4. T.
5. T.

#### Crossword puzzle

*Across*

2. Dizziness.
3. Bacoflen.
4. Chlorphensin.
6. Spasticity.
8. Dantrolene.
9. Pregnancy.

*Down*

10. Methocarbamol.
1. Massage.
5. Orphenadrine.
7. Diazepam.

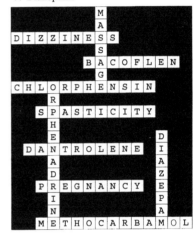

#### Review questions

1. d.
2. a.
3. b.
4. c.
5. d.
6. b.
7. d.
8. d.
9. c.
10. d.

## CHAPTER 14
### Anesthetics

#### Matching exercise: terms and concepts

1. B.
2. A.
3. E.
4. C.
5. I.
6. K.
7. H.
8. G.
9. D.
10. F.
11. L.
12. M.
13. N.
14. P.
15. R.

**Word scramble**

1. ETHRANE
2. FORANE
3. ALFENTA
4. INNOVAR
5. PAVULON
6. ANECTINE
7. METUBINE
8. SULFENTA
9. VERSED
10. BREVITAL

**Review questions**

1. a.
2. b.
3. c.
4. c.
5. b.
6. d.
7. a.
8. d.
9. c.
10. b.

## CHAPTER 15
### Alcohol and Other Drug Abuse

**Matching exercise: terms and concepts**

1. B.
2. C.
3. E.
4. G.
5. A.
6. F.
7. I.
8. D.
9. H.
10. J.

11. K.
12. M.
13. L.
14. O.
15. N.

**Nursing diagnosis**

*Nursing Diagnoses*

1. Alteration in nutrition: malnutrition and vitamin deficiencies.
2. High risk for violence related to altered thought process.
3. Decreased cardiac output associated with fluid volume excess.
4. High risk for injury related to bleeding.

*Assessment Data*

1. Lab studies assess for anemia and electrolyte imbalances. Assess client for signs/symptoms of a deficiency.
2. Assess client for impaired motor coordination, poor task performance, hypo-/hyperactivity.
3. Assess heart sounds and lung sounds, ECGs. Assess lab studies, serum albumin levels.
4. Assess platelet count and clotting studies.

*Nursing Interventions*

1. Administer folic acid and thiamine, vitamin $B_{12}$.
2. Administer Librium. Decrease environmental stimuli. Teach non-drug coping techniques.
3. q4h vs, peripheral pulses, administer diuretics if appropriate. I&O daily weights.
4. Observe client for bruising.

*DEFINE:*

ALCOHOLISM: a chronic, progressive, potentially fatal disease; characterized by physical dependence and physiologic changes related to the ingestion of alcohol.

PSYCHOLOGICAL DEPENDENCE: feelings of satisfaction and pleasure from taking a drug.

PHYSICAL DEPENDENCE: physiologic adaption to chronic drug use resulting in uncomfortable symptoms when the drug is stopped.

**Review questions**

1. c.
2. b.
3. d.
4. c.
5. c.
6. d.
7. c.
8. c.
9. b.
10. a.

## CHAPTER 16
### Central Nervous System Stimulants

**Complete the following sentences**

1. narcolepsy; ADD (attention deficit disorder).
2. a rare disorder characterized.
3. children; hyperactivity, a short attention span, difficulty in completing assigned tasks, restlessness and impulsive behavior.
4. mood elevation and increased mental alertness. heart rate; blood pressure; mydriasis; gastrointestinal motility. tolerance and dependence.
5. respiration. seizures.
6. mental alertness; drowsiness.
7. cardiovascular disease, anxiety, agitated states, glaucoma, hyperthyroidism.
8. (Dexedrine); narcolepsy.
9. (Ritalin); 6–8.
10. (Dopram), 5–10.

**Chapter 14 Word Scramble**

11. analgesia. migrane headaches.
12. neonates.
13. caffeine intake.
14. caffeine.
15. weight; height.
16. excessive CNS stimulation, cardio-vascular, gastrointestinal.

## Review questions

1. a.
2. d.
3. c.
4. b.
5. b.
6. a.
7. b.
8. c.
9. a.
10. b.

## CHAPTER 17
## Physiology of the Autonomic Nervous System

### Autonomic Nervous System Chart

(See below)

### True or false

1. T.
2. T.
3. F.  .
4. F.
5. F.
6. F.

### Review questions

1. b.
2. a.
3. c.
4. a.
5. b.
6. b.
7. d.
8. b.
9. d.
10. c.

## CHAPTER 18
## Adrenergic Drugs

### Matching exercise: terms and concepts

1. C.
2. D.
3. A.
4. F.
5. E.
6. B.
7. I.
8. G.
9. H.
10. J.

### True or false

1  T.
2. F.
3. F.
4. T.
5. T.
6. T.
7. F.
8. F.
9. T.
10. T.

### Sentence correction

1. Isoproterenol (Isuprel).
2. Anaphylactic.
3. Allergens.
4. Acidosis.
5. 30.
6. Epinephrine.
7. Stokes–Adams.
8. Phenylephrine.
9. Tachycardia.
10. Under.
11. Blood pressure.
12. Rebound nasal congestion.
13. Urinary output.
14. Increase.
15. Hypotension and shock.

### Review questions

1. b.
2. a.
3. d.
4. c.
5. d.
6. c.
7. a.
8  c.
9. c.
10. b.

## CHAPTER 19
## Antiadrenergic Drugs

### Matching exercise: terms and concepts

1. E.
2. F.
3. A.
4. D.
5. B.
6. C.
7. I.
8. G.
9. H.
10. J.

### True or false

1. T.
2. F.
3. T.
4. T.
5. F.

### Beta receptor sites

*Part A*

1. Nerve ending.
2. Receptor site.
3. Myocardial or other cell tissue.
4. Beta adrenergic blocking drug.
5. Epinephrine and norepinephrine.

### Sentence correction

1. Propranolol (Inderal).
2. Selective.
3. Supraventricular tachycardia.
4. Timolol (Timoptic).
5. Propranolol (Inderal).
6. Labetalol (Trandate).
7. Atenolol (Tenormin).
8. Nonselective.
9. Propranolol (Inderal).
10. Alpha adrenergic blocking agents.
11. Decreasing.
12. Beta$_1$.
13. Bradycardia.
14. Lipid.
15. Decreased.

### Review questions

1. d.
2. b.
3. a.
4. c.
5. b.
6. a.
7. b.
8. d.
9. b.
10. c.

## CHAPTER 20
## Cholinergic Drugs

1. parasympathetic.
2. a. decreased.
   b. increased.
   c. relaxation of.
   d. increased.
   e. increased.
   f. increased.
   g. constriction of.

## Chapter 17 Chart

| PARA-SYMPATHETIC | Location | SYMPATHETIC | | | |
|---|---|---|---|---|---|
| | | alpha$^1$ | alpha$^2$ | beta$^1$ | beta$^2$ |
| dilation | blood vessels | constriction | | | |
| decreases force | heart | | | increases force | |
| bronchoconstriction | lungs | | | | bronchodilation |
| increases motility | GI | | | | decreases motility |
| constriction | eye | dilation | | | |
| | liver | | | | glycogenolysis |
| | platelet | | aggregation | | |

**Match the drug with its action**
1. D.
2. A.
3. B.
4. C.
5. E.

**True or false**
1. T.
2. F.
3. F.
4. T.
5. T.

**Review questions**
1. b.
2. c.
3. a.
4. b.
5. a.
6. d.
7. a.
8. c.
9. d.
10. d.

# CHAPTER 21
## Anticholinergic Drugs

**Complete the following sentences**
1. acetylcholine; parasympathetic.
2. a. CNS stimulation followed by CNS depression.
   b. slows heart rate.
   c. bronchodilation and decreased respiratory tract secretion.
   d. antispasmodic effect in GI tract.
   e. mydriasis and cycloplegia.
   f. increased secretion of sweat glands, relaxation of ureters and bladder, relaxation of smooth muscle of gall bladder and bile ducts.
3. peptic ulcer disease, gastritis, pylorospasm, diverticulitis, ileitis, and ulcerative colitis.
4. examination; surgery; mydriatic and cycloplegic.
5. increase.
6. inhalation.
7. increase bladder capacity.
8. respiratory secretions; vagal stimulation.
9. prostatic hypertrophy, glaucoma, tachyarrhythmias, myocardial infarction, CHF.
10. prototype PO; IM, IV, SC, topically; inhalation.
11. spasm; increased secretion, increased motility.
12. motion sickness. patch; 72.
13. Trihexyphenidyl, Parkinsonism. extrapyramidal reactions.
14. Benztropine; acute dystonic reactions.
15. dysuria, urgency, frequency, pain.
16. (Ditropan); bladder capacity; frequency.
17. blurred vision, confusion, heat stroke, constipation, urinary retention, hallucinations, psychotic-like symptoms.

**True or false**
1. F.
2. T.
3. F.
4. F.
5. F.

**Matching exercise**
1. C.
2. D.
3. A.
4. B.
5. E.

**Review questions**
1. d.
2. c.
3. c.
4. b.
5. a.
6. b.
7. c.
8. a.
9. b.
10. d.

# CHAPTER 22
## Physiology of the Endocrine System

**Matching exercise: terms and concepts**
1. D.
2. E.
3. F.
4. I.
5. J.
6. A.
7. B.
8. G.
9. C.
10. H.

**True or false**
1. T.
2. F.
3. T.
4. F.
5. T.

**Review questions**
1. c.
2. a.
3. c.
4. a.
5. a.
6. d.
7. b.
8. c.
9. a.
10. b.

# CHAPTER 23
## Hypothalamic and Pituitary Hormones

**Matching exercise: terms and concepts**
1. M.
2. G.
3. A.
4. D.
5. J.
6. I.
7. N.
8. H.

9. B.
10. C.
11. E.
12. K.
13. F.
14. L.
15. O.

**Review questions**
1. c.
2. b.
3. a.
4. c.
5. d.
6. d.
7. a.
8. a.
9. a.
10. d.

# CHAPTER 24
## Corticosteroids

**True or false**
1. F.
2. F.
3. F.
4. T.
5. T.
6. T.
7. T.
8. T.
9. F.
10. T.
11. T.
12. T.
13. T.
14. T.
15. F.

**Undesirable effects of drug administration**
1.
2. X
3. X
4. X
5. X
6. X
7.
8. X
9. X
10. X
11.
12. X
13. X
14. X
15. X
16. X
17. X
18.
19.
20. X
21. X
22. X
23.
24. X

## Word scramble

1. VANCERIL
2. CELESTONE
3. FLORINEF
4. AEROBID
5. ARISTOSPAN
6. CORTEF
7. MEDROL
8. STERANE
9. CORTONE
10. DECADRON
11. HALDRONE
12. ARISTOCORT
13. HYDELTRASOL
14. DELTASONE

## Review questions

1. b.
2. c.
3. b.
4. a.
5. c.
6. c.
7. b.
8. d.
9. b.
10. b.

## CHAPTER 25
### Thyroid and Antithyroid Drugs

### Complete the following sentences

1. Iodine.
2. metabolism.
3. growth and development.
4. myxedema; variable depending on amount of thyroid tissue and hormone production.
5. nervousness, emotional instability, restlessness, anxiety, insomnia, hyperactive reflexes.
6. tachycardia, fever, dehydration, heart failure.
7. antithyroid drugs, radioactive iodine, surgery, a combination of methods.
8. Synthroid; 1. 0.1–0.2.
9. hyperthyroidism.
10. propranolol (Inderal).
11. 0.08–0.20 mg/100 ml; 5–12 µg/100 ml.
12. 12.
13. height, weight.
14. 100.

### Nursing diagnosis

*Nursing Diagnoses*

1. Altered nutrition: less than body requirement.
2. Altered bowel elimination: diarrhea.
3. Altered comfort related to hypermetabolic state.
4. Knowledge deficit: related to drug therapy.
5. Altered cardiac output.

*Assessment Data*

1. Assess weight.
2. Assess for electrolyte imbalance.

3. Assess nutrition
4. Assess client's knowledge of medication.
5. Monitor vital signs. Observe for symptoms of CHF.

*Related Interventions*

1. Provide extra calories.
2. Instruct to increase fluids. Instruct to avoid foods that cause diarrhea.
3. Instruct to take cool baths and wear lightweight clothing. Instruct to rest.
4. Instruct client regarding antithyroid drugs.
5. Administer propranolol (Inderal) if appropriate.

*DEFINE:*

GOITER: enlargement of the thyroid gland resulting from iodine deficiency.
CRETINISM: occurs as the result of a poorly functioning thyroid gland and results in poor growth and development in children.
MYXEDEMA: a condition resulting from hypofunctioning of the thyroid gland.
THYROID STORM: a complication of thyrotoxicosis; symptoms of which include severe tachycardia, fever, dehydration, heart failure, and coma.

### Review questions

1. c.
2. a.
3. c.
4. c.
5. d.
6. b.
7. a
8. d.
9. b.
10. d.

## Chapter 24 Word Scramble

```
A P P L H E X N O T H S B H Y P O F T I L C L C E
B F G H D J K A D R E N E R G I C E N B E C T A Z
C O L A E N E C M R A I S S A N L L X Q K O V Z S
D E A N L V C D N C H T N H X Y Z T I P L R D N E
E G G H T D R O E O N I R Y L A R N V R H T L P O
F O N T A D I L N C A Y Y D O D A V P P J O F N V
A N L E S C B R E I K X F E H T G N A E B N O S B
R I F L O R I N E F L U A L A C A A I D A E U K L
O E E U N R E T O R P M X T T O S H R F R N O H A
Y P X C E L E S T O N E D R K B B L K A O T L R N
A J R E C L N O N O T D H A R I S T O C O R T S B
H Y P O F T I L C L C R E S F G H H J N K K A D R
E N E R G I C E L N B O E O T D A Z O L O L A N E
C M R A I S S I A N E L L L X E K V Z S X C W C A
H L P O D I R L A U D I D N A C A Y Y O D A U P J
R I L U A E A C A A I D A V H A L D R O N E H A P
D K B E C L A O T L R N A Y J D R E C L N O S T Y
M P E N A M B E R E C V A S G R O N I Q P P F E N
T A A E R O B I D N Y L K I G O N L O K C T K X T
G V A A N G A R I S T O S P A N T A P E S C O R N
I U O U S A L E T M O D T I I B T U D H T R P P L
A S O N B S O R P H Y D R O C O C O R T E F I O N
C W A C I N U C N K I X O P T O R I T A R N G I N
Y B P I X K U N L S I N E T A X A A Y B A I D L E
S F N D N S V D F H C I A N I G E M O R N P H A N
K O N M H L O R Z I D E G D E P E R R T E S P L O
```

## CHAPTER 26
### Hormones That Regulate Calcium and Phosphorus Metabolism

#### Complete the following sentences

1. parathyroid hormone, calcitonin.
2. up; down.
3. a. increases bone breakdown or reabsorption.
   b. increase absorption of calcium from food.
   c. increase reabsorption of calcium in renal tubules.
4. lowers bone; serum; rapid; short. long-term.
5. foods; exposure to sunlight. serum calcium levels; increasing; mobilizing calcium from bone.
6. (Rocaltrol); daily.
7. calcium; phosphorus.
8. 8.5 mg–10 mg/100 ml.
9. a. cell membrane permeability and function.
   b. nerve cell excitability and transmission of function.
   c. muscle cell excitation and coupling.
   d. blood coagulation and platelet adhesion.
   e. hormone and enzyme activities.
10. milk, vegetables (broccoli) (spinach) (kale) (mustard greens), seafood (clams) (oysters).
11. Vitamin D deficiency, high-fat diet, presence of oxalic acid from beet greens and chard, alkalinity of intestinal secretions, diarrhea.
12. a. is an essential component of DNA, RNA and nucleic acid.
    b. combines with fatty acids to form phospholipids which are required in the structure of all cell membranes.
    c. forms phosphate buffer system.
    d. is necessary for cell utilization of glucose.
    e. is necessary for proper function of B vitamins.
13. neuromuscular irritability; tetany.
14. increases.
15. Chvostek's; Trousseau's.
16. 30 minutes before.
17. vitamin D.
18. steroids (Prednisone), calcitonin, mithromycin, phosphates, antacids.
19. Cancer.
20. Irreversible damage; impairment of function.
21. lowers.
22. Lasix increases.
23. vitamin D; decreasing.
24. blocking resorption from bone; bone marrow depression.
25. reabsorption of calcium in renal tubules.
26. 3000–4000 ml/day; kidney stones.

#### True or false

1. T.
2. F.
3. T.
4. F.
5. T.

#### Review questions

1. c.
2. d.
3. b.
4. b.
5. a.
6. d.
7. c.
8. a.
9. b.
10. c.

## CHAPTER 27
### Antidiabetic Agents

#### Specify Increases or Decreases

1. Increases.
2. Decreases.
3. Decreases.
4. Increases.
5. Increases.
6. Decreases.
7. Decreases.

#### Matching exercise: terms and concepts

1. C.
2. D.
3. F.
4. H.
5. E.
6. I.
7. J.
8. K.
9. M.
10. N.

#### True or false

1. T.
2. T.
3. F.
4. T.
5. F.
6. F.
7. T.
8. F.
9. T.
10. T.
11. T.
12. F.

#### Crossword puzzle

*Across*

5. Lipid.
7. Beef.
10. Acetohexamide.
12. Isophane.

*Down*

1. Salicylates.
2. Hypoglycemia.
3. Lipodystrophy.
4. Glyburide.
6. Ketoacidosis.
8. Tolazmide.
9. Glipizide.
11. Human.

#### Review questions

1. a.
2. b.
3. d.
4. a.
5. d.
6. a.
7. d.
8. c.
9. a.
10. d.

## CHAPTER 28
### Estrogens, Progestins, and Oral Contraceptives

#### True or false

1. T.
2. F.
3. T.
4. T.
5. T.
6. F.
7. T.
8. F.
9. T.
10. F.
11. T.
12. T.
13. T.
14. F.
15. T.

#### Name that drug

1. estradiol transdermal system (Estraderm).
2. dienestrol (DV).
3. DES (Stilbestrol).
4. conjugated estrogen (Premarin).
5. estradiol valerate (Delestrogen).
6. estradiol cypionate (Depo-Estradiol).
7. hydroxy progesterone caproate (Delalutin).
8. medroxy progesterone (Depo-Provera).
9. Premarin.
10. estrogen (Premarin).
11. oral contraceptives.
12. estropipate (Ogen).
13. hydroxy progesterone caproate (Delautin)
14. Micronor Nor-Q.D. (Overette).
15. Neomycin.

**Review questions**

1. c.
2. d.
3. a.
4. c.
5. b.
6. c.
7. a.
8. a.
9. d.
10. c.

## CHAPTER 29
### Androgens and Anabolic Steroids

**Circle the correct answer**

1. increase.
2. increases, decreases.
3. increased.
4. decreases.
5. increased.
6. increase.
7. decreases.
8. increased
9. decreased.
10. increase.
11. increase.
12. increases.
13. decrease.
14. increase.
15. increase.

**Crossword puzzle**

*Across*

4. Halotestin.
7. Danzanol.
8. Testosterone.
9. Oxandrolone.
10. Electrolyte.

*Down*

1. Epiphyseal.
2. Insulin.
3. Gonadotropic.
5. Exogenous.
6. Testoject.

```
                              D
                              A
        I N S U L I N         N
                              A
E L E C T R O L Y T E         Z
X           E                 O
O     E P I P H Y S E A L
G           T
E           O
N     H A L O T E S T I N
O           T
U     T E S T O J E C T
S           R
  G O N A D O T R O P I C
            N
O X A N D R O L O N E
```

**Review questions**

1. b.
2. d.
3. c.
4. d.
5. d.
6. b.
7. c.
8. b.

9. b.
10. b.

## CHAPTER 30
### Nutritional Products, Anorexiants, and Digestants

**Fill in the blank**

1. P.
2. W, F.
3. C.
4. P.
5. W.
6. C.
7. W.
8. C.
9. F.
10. F.

**True or false**

1. F.
2. T.
3. F.
4. T.
5. F.
6. T.
7. F.
8. F.
9. T.
10. F.

**Matching exercise**

1. C.
2. B.
3. F.
4. G.
5. E.
6. A.
7. D.

**Complete the following sentences**

1. D5W; 170.
2. 20, 50. hypertonic.
3. 550.
4. water.
5. hypertonic; increase.
6. protein; calories.
7. essential fatty acids; centrally or peripherally.
8. tube placement.
9. 500 ml.
10. 1000.

**Review questions**

1. a.
2. d.
3. b.
4. c.
5. d.
6. b.
7. c.
8. c.
9. a.
10. b.

## CHAPTER 31
### Vitamins

**Matching exercise: terms and concepts**

1. D.
2. F.
3. H.
4. J.
5. L.
6. A.
7. B.
8. E.
9. I.
10. C.
11. G.
12. M.
13. K.

**Name the deficiency/excess**

1. Vitamin A def.
2. Vitamin K def.
3. Biotin def.
4. Pyridoxine (vitamin $B_6$ def.)
5. Vitamin C excess, vitamin A def.
6. Severe thiamine def.
7. Vitamin B def.
8. Severe vitamin C def.
9. Folic acid def., thiamine def.
10. Vitamin A excess.
11. Vitamin C def.
12. Riboflavin def.
13. Niacin def.
14. Vitamin C excess.
15. Vitamin $B_{12}$ def.
16. Vitamin $B_{12}$ def.
17. Vitamin K def.
18. Vitamin A excess.
19. Folic acid def., thiamine def.
20. Vitamin C def.

**Review questions**

1. c.
2. d.
3. b.
4. b.
5. a.
6. a.
7. d.
8. a.
9. a.
10. c.

## CHAPTER 32
### Minerals and Electrolytes

**Matching exercise: terms and concepts**

1. G.
2. F.
3. D.
4. H.
5. M.
6. I.
7. A.
8. K.
9. B.
10. P.
11. C.
12. E.
13. J.
14. L.
15. O.

## Name that imbalance

1. Hyperkalemia.
2. Zinc deficiency.
3. Hypernatremia.
4. Hypercupremia.
5. Hyperkalemia.
6. Chromium deficiency.
7. Hypokalemia.
8. Hypocupremia.
9. Hyponatremia, hypomagnesemia, hypochloremia.
10. Hemochromatosis.
11. Hypernatremia.
12. Iron deficiency, hypocupremia.
13. Hyponatremia.
14. Hypermagnesemia.
15. Hypokalemia.
16. Hyperchloremia.
17. Hypochloremia, hypocalcemia.
18. Hyperkalemia.
19. Hypomagnesemia.
20. Hypermagnesemia.

## Review questions

1. d.
2. a.
3. b.
4. a.
5. c.
6. d.
7. b.
8. d.
9. a.
10. c.

## CHAPTER 33
## General Characteristics of Anti-infective Drugs

## Complete the following sentences

1. a. breaks in skin.
   b. impaired blood supply.
   c. neutropenia.
   d. malnutrition.
   e. poor hygiene.
   f. suppression of normal flora.
   g. suppression of immune system.
   h. diabetes mellitus.
   i. advanced age.
2. nosocomial.

3. antibacterial, antiviral, antifungal.
4. bactericidal.
5. bacteriostatic.
6. 7–10.
7. reduced. creatinine.
8. aminoglycosides.
9. 1–2 hrs; 8.
10. hypersensitivity, superinfection, phlebiti, gastrointestinal symptoms.
11. a. stomatitis.
    b. diarrhea.
    c. monilial vaginitis.
    d. new signs and symptoms.
    e. recurrent signs and symptoms.

## Review questions

1. b.
2. c.
3. b.
4. a.
5. a.
6. b.
7. a.
8. b.
9. c.
10. d.

## CHAPTER 34
## Penicillins

## Complete the following sentences

1. a. streptococcal pharyngitis.
   b. pneumococcal pneumonia.
   c. gonorrhea.
   d. syphilis.
2. dental, surgical procedures.
3. Cloxacillin, Dicloxacillin, Methicillin, Nafcillin, Oxacillin.
4. Ampicillin.
5. urinary tract, biliary tract, respiratory, ear.
6. Ampicillin; Sulbactam.
7. Carbenicillin, Ticarcillin, Mezlocillin, Piperacillin.
8. rash, hives, swelling, difficulty in breathing.
9. Unipen; IV or IM; 4–6, 50–100
10. seriousness.
11. increase; blocking renal excretion.
12. 50–100; 30–60.

## Word scramble

1. GEOPEN
2. AMOXIL
3. TEGOPEN
4. UNIPEN
5. TICAR
6. AZLIN
7. MEZLIN
8. PIPRACIL
9. STAPHCILLIN
10. DYNAPEN
11. PROSTAPHIN
12. AUGMENTIN
13. VERSAPEN
14. COACTIN

## Review questions

1. a.
2. a.
3. c.
4. d.
5. b.
6. a.
7. c.
8. a.
9. a.
10. b.

## CHAPTER 35
## Cephalosporins

## Complete the following sentences

1. bacterial cell walls.
2. gram pos. and gram neg. organisms
3. first, second, third.
4. a. surgical prophylaxis.
   b. respiratory tract infections.
   c. skin infections.
   d. soft tissue and bone infections.
   e. urinary tract.
   f. bloodstream infections.
5. skin rash, drug fever, eosinophilia.
6. Keflex; Velosef; Kefzol; Ancef.
7. Ceclor.
8. not readily reached by other drugs; immunosuppressed.
9. Cefotan; Rocephin.
10. 6; thrombophlebitis; 1.
11. renal failure; 50.

## Chapter 34 Word Scramble

12. increased BUN, increased serum creatinine, casts in the urine.
13. Mandol, Cefobid, Moxam; kill intestinal bacteria that normally produce vitamin K or prevent activation of prothrombin.
14. aminoglycosides; renal toxicity.
15. diarrhea, especially if it contains blood, pus, or mucus.

### Crossword puzzle

*Across*

2. Ceftriaxone.
4. Cefoperazone.
6. Moxalactam.
7. Prosthetic.
9. Penicillin.
10. Cerebrospinal.

*Down*

1. Cefoxitin.
3. Tetracyclines.
4. Cefazolin.
5. Cephalexin.
8. Renal.

### Review questions

1. c.
2. c.
3. d.
4. a.
5. b.
6. c.
7. b.
8. d.
9. b.
10. d.

## CHAPTER 36
### Aminoglycosides

### Complete the following sentences

1. gram-negative.
2. serious and life-threatening infections.
3. suppress intestinal bacteria; ammonia.
4. nephrotoxic, ototoxic, renal impairment.
5. resistant to other aminoglycosides; 15 mg.
6. 275.
7. oral, topical, eye, ear, skin.
8. a. check renal function studies.
   b. assess for hearing impairment.
   c. analyze medications, assess other drugs that may be nephrotoxic.
   d. weigh client.

9. a. serum drug levels; renal function studies.
   b. at least 2000–3000 ml daily.
10. 30–60; trough, 10–12; 2.
11. diuretics.
12. 10.

### Review questions

1. a.
2. a.
3. b.
4. b.
5. b.
6. d.
7. b.
8. d.
9. c.
10. c.

## CHAPTER 37
### Tetracyclines

### Complete the following sentences

1. gram positive, gram-negative, rickettsiae, mycoplasmas and protazo spirochetes and others.
2. penicillins, cephalosporins.
3. a. urethral, endocervical, or rectal infections caused by chlamydia.
   b. for PID and STD with other antimicrobials.
   c. acne.
   d. pleural effusions.
   e. treat inappropriate secretion of ADH.
   f. in patients allergic to penicillin.
   g. prophylactically for travelers' diarrhea.
4. have renal failure; less than 8 years of age.
5. mottling of tooth enamel, may interfere with bone growth.
6. 1 hr before meals.
7. metallic ions.
8. sunlight; a sunburn or skin reaction.
9. superinfection.
10. renal insufficiency; pregnant.
11. methoxyflurane, sulfonamides.
12. decrease.
13. nausea, vomiting, diarrhea, skin rash, perineal.
14. milk.

### Review questions

1. d.
2. a.
3. c.
4. d.
5. c.
6. c.
7. b.
8. a.
9. d.
10. a.

## CHAPTER 38
### Macrolides

### Complete the following sentences

1. bacteriostatic; high.
2. a. suppression of intestinal bacteria.
   b. Legionnaires' disease.
   c. infections caused by mycoplasma pneumoniae.
   d. prevention of whooping cough.

   e. elimination of the diphtheria carrier.
   f. substitute for penicillin.
3. have pre-existing liver disease.
4. gram-positive organisms.
5. renal faliure.
6. suppress normal flora of the bowel.
7. 1 hour before or 2 hours after a meal.
8. an empty.
9. nausea, vomiting, diarrhea.
10. nausea, vomiting, abdominal cramps, fever, leukocytosis, abnormal liver function, and possibly jaundice.

### True or false

1. T.
2. F.
3. F.
4. F.
5. F.

### Review questions

1. a.
2. b.
3. b.
4. b.
5. d.
6. d.
7. c.
8. a.
9. d.
10. c.

## CHAPTER 39
### Miscellaneous Anti-infectives

### Complete the following sentences

1. Azactam; gram-negative.
2. Azactam;
   a. does not appear to cause kidney or hearing damage.
   b. preserves normal gram-positive and anaerobic flora.
3. Primaxin; organisms resistant to other drugs.
4. Noroxin; UTIs.
5. Cipro; a wide variety of infections.
6. Chloromycetin; typhoid fever; serious infections.
7. Coly-Mycin; ear infections.
8. Trobicin; gonococcal infections.
9. Vancomycin; severe; nephrotoxic.
10. a. newer beta lactams.
    b. quinolones.
    c. vancomycin.

### Review questions

1. b.
2. c.
3. c.
4. d.
5. a.
6. a.
7. a.
8. c.
9. d.
10. a.

## CHAPTER 40
### Sulfonamides and Urinary Antiseptics

### Complete the following sentences

1. *E. coli*, proteus, *Klebsiella*.
2. burn wound infections, ocular, vaginal, soft tissue infections.
3. having had a hypersensitivity reaction to sulfonamides or diuretics or antidiabetic agents, renal failure, late pregnancy, lactation, children under 2; salicylates.
4. (Cinobac); gram-negative.
5. (Mandelamine); (Hiprex); acidification. Ascorbic acid.
6. (Furadantin, Macrodantin), gram-negative, gram positive.
7. (Pyridium); dysuria, burning, frequency, urgency. orange red.
8. 1200–1500.
9. alkaline.
10. acidic.
11. (Bactrim), (Septra); severe skin reactions, bone marrow depression, folic acid deficiency.

### True or false

1. F.
2. T.
3. F.
4. F.
5. T.

### Review questions

1. a.
2. c.
3. d.
4. c.
5. a.
6. a.
7. a.
8. c.
9. b.
10. d.

## CHAPTER 41
### Antitubercular Drugs

### Complete the following sentence

1. 6.
2. INH, Rifampin, Pyrazinamide, Streptomycin.
3. organisms are resistant to primary drugs.
4. skin test.
5. with hepatic disease; to the drug; who are pregnant.
6. body secretions, red-orange.
7. body weight.
8. para-amino salicylic acid (PAS), Capreomycin, Cycloserine, Ethionamide.
9. liver function studies.
10. with food.
11. 1 hr before or 2 hrs after a meal.
12. hepatotoxicity.
13. nephrotoxicity.
14. a. GI problems.
    b. yellow sclera, dark urine, clay-colored stools.
    c. changes in hearing or vision.
    d. numbness or tingling.
    e. dizziness, drowsiness, skin rash or fever.

15. fever, tachycardia, anorexia, malaise, 3rd, 8th.

### Review questions

1. d.
2. a.
3. d.
4. b.
5. b.
6. c.
7. b.
8. c.
9. c.
10. c.

## CHAPTER 42
### Antiviral Drugs

### True or false

1. F.
2. F.
3. T.
4. F.
5. T.
6. T.
7. F.
8. T.
9. F.
10. F.
11. F.
12. T.
13. T.
14. T.
15. T.

### Review questions

1. d.
2. a.
3. b.
4. c.
5. c.

6. d.
7. b.
8. c.
9. c.
10. c.

## CHAPTER 43
### Antifungal Drugs

### Matching exercise: terms and concepts

1. A.
2. G.
3. F.
4. J.
5. I.
6. C.
7. H.
8. E.
9. B.
10. D.
11. O.
12. K.
13. M.
14. N.
15. Q.

### Word scramble

1. FULVICIN
2. ANCOBON
3. SPECTAZOLE
4. DESENEX
5. TINACTIN
6. MYCOSTATIN
7. NATACYN
8. MONISTAT
9. NIZORAL
10. LOTRIMIN
11. LOPROX
12. AKRINOL

### Chapter 43 Word Scramble

```
D A R D R S C O P B U T A N T I A A D M P H E T N
T E A D A E I O A N T I P A R A I C G R A N T I I
A H S P E C T A Z O L E H Y P S S Y M P A M I N C
C R A E R O D N A A D R E N E P I A S I S M B A T
D X T I N A C T I N R P I N E F N A G R E N E N A
C I G A R E P P Y S O I M I M O N I S T A T M P E
N L O P R O X A M M E A N I T I N A R E V O L A P
D I A T L E V O P H E D D N C G I D N E A R D A H
N E D E D O N I A N T I A I L E A I E D E P E N I
S A R I N U B A T A C I V R E N I L O H C I T N A
I I A A B O S A H I S L P N I N E R S S T I T D U
I M M A D S U M O Y U E I I I P E O T N C I G R T
P N S N I I D I M F E R P P I N S R I C A I C A O
N E I T M S A P I C H E C E O P E C G D A I B C A
S Y M C H A A T M P P H E L O T R I M I N E S I U
E L N C O T E P E C O T I I T O L I Y E C Y C B T
I N E I H T O N T L V I N P T I A N C H O C M E O
A L I E Z I I N I E E H O G A D R O N B L I N N
P E T P E O H N C R L A G R N R O G S C O T D I O
N I A H E P R D E P H R N T E C N U T A N T R I M
C R N R A R P A K R I N O L I C N T A I T A I S I
T A O E G A N G L I A D E N A M A A T O S I A H C
T N A I S C O P O L A M I N E P N B I A M O S O M
N T C W P H E D R I A S N A T A C Y N R E N I M A
A I I H A P P R I O D L N I I F I R T A S I S M N
N C T P O P H I A S R D E S F A E P I N E P I N E
I C I G R E N I L O H C I T N A P H E D R E I S T
```

**Review questions**

1. d.
2. c.
3. b.
4. b.
5. a.
6. c.
7. d.
8. a.
9. d.
10. a.

## CHAPTER 44
### Antiparasitics

**True or false**

1. T.
2. T.
3. T.
4. F.
5. F.
6. T.
7. T.
8. F.
9. T.
10. F.
11. T.
12. F.
13. T.
14. T.
15. T.

**Review questions**

1. a.
2. b.
3. a.
4. c.
5. c.
6. a.
7. a.
8. b.
9. c.
10. d.

## CHAPTER 45
### Physiology of the Immune System

**Matching exercise: terms and concepts**

1. D.
2. A.
3. H.
4. J.
5. B.
6. C.
7. E.
8. O.
9. L.
10. F.
11. N.
12. I.
13. G.
14. K.
15. M.

**Review questions**

1. a.
2. a.
3. d.
4. b.
5. d.

6. c.
7. d.
8. a.
9. d.
10. a.

## CHAPTER 46
### Immunizing Agents

**Complete the following sentences**

1. protection or resistance to a disease.
2. antigen; antibody formation; brief; long term.
3. antibodies, a few weeks or months.
4. febrile illness, impaired cellular immunity, those on steroids or receiving immunosuppressant drugs, leukemia, pregnancy.
5. 10.
6. a. cholera.
   b. smallpox.
   c. yellow fever.
7. health-care workers and renal transplant patients, dialysis patients, multiple blood transfusions, immunosuppressed, homosexual males.
8. 2 months, 4 months, 6 months, 18 months, 4–5 years.
9. 12–15 months.
10. Influenza.
11. temperature.
12. epinephrine (Adrenalin).
13. tenderness, redness; Tylenol.
14. Paralysis (Guillain-Barré syndrome).
15. serum sickness; days, weeks.

**Review questions**

1. c.
2. a.
3. d.
4. c.
5. d.
6. d.
7. d.
8. b.
9. d.
10. c.

## CHAPTER 47
### Immunostimulants

**Matching exercise: terms and concepts**

1. B.
2. D.
3. F.
4. H.
5. I.
6. G.
7. E.
8. A.
9. J.
10. K.

**True or false**

1. T.
2. F.
3. F.
4. T.
5. T.

**Crossword puzzle**

*Across*

1. Aldesleukin.
3. Interferon.
4. Neutrophil.
6. Condylomata.
8. Filgrastim.
9. Leukopenia.

*Down*

2. Sargramostim.
5. BCG.
7. Solid.

**Review questions**

1. d.
2. b.
3. b.
4. b.
5. b.
6. c.
7. a.
8. d.
9. c.
10. b.

## CHAPTER 48
### Immunosuppressants

**True or false**

1. T.
2. F.
3. F.
4. F.
5. T.
6. T.
7. T.
8. F.
9. F.
10. F.
11. T.
12. T.
13. F.
14. F.
15. T.

**Review questions**

1. d.
2. c.
3. c.
4. a.
5. b.
6. d.
7. a.
8. c.
9. c.
10. d.

## CHAPTER 49
### Physiology of the Respiratory System

**Matching exercise: terms and concepts**

1. D.
2. F.
3. G.
4. I.
5. C.
6. J.
7. K.
8. L.
9. B.
10. N.
11. S.
12. R.
13. V.
14. X.
15. Z.

**Review questions**

1. a.
2. a.
3. a.
4. c.
5. b.
6. c.
7. d.
8. c.
9. b.
10. d.

## CHAPTER 50
### Bronchodilating and Antiasthmatic Drugs

**Matching exercise: terms and concepts**

1. B.
2. C.
3. D.
4. A.

**Complete the following sentences**

1. a. respiratory infections.
   b. odors.
   c. smoke.
   d. cold air.
   e. exercise.
   f. emotional upsets.
   g. tartrazine.
   h. fumes.
   i. drugs.
2. Adrenalin; acute attack of bronchospasm; 5 minutes.
3. Proventil; orally, inhalation.
4. Atrovent; 15. cough, nervousness, nausea, GI upset, headache, dizziness.
5. (Beclovent) (Vanceril), (Azmacort); inhalation.
6. short, long
7. Intal; allergic asthma, exercise induced asthma.
8. tachypnea, dyspnea, use of accessory muscles, hypoxia.
9. confusion, restlessness, anxiety, ↑BP, ↑pulse.
10. 2000–3000; thin their secretions. nervousness, insomnia.
11. a. shake before use.
    b. remove cap.
    c. exhale fully.

d. insert inhaler, form a tight seal.
e. inhale, depress inhaler.
f. hold breath.
g. wait 3–5 minutes before 2nd inhalation.
h. rinse mouth piece.
12. The bronchodilator.
13. fungal infection of the mouth and throat.

**True or false**

1. F.
2. T.
3. T.
4. F.
5. F.
6. T.

**Review questions**

1. c.
2. d.
3. a.
4. b.
5. b.
6. b.
7. d.
8. a.
9. d.
10. d.

## CHAPTER 51
### Antihistamines

**Matching exercise: terms and concepts**

1. B.
2. C.
3. E.
4. G.
5. A.
6. F.
7. H.
8. J.
9. I.
10. D.
11. L.
12. N.

**Review questions**

1. c.
2. d.
3. c.
4. d.
5. c.
6. b.
7. c.
8. a.
9. d.
10. b.

## CHAPTER 52
### Nasal Decongestants, Antitussives, Mucolytics, and Cold Remedies

**Complete the following sentences**

1. nasal decongestants.
2. profuse discharge from the nose.
3. cough.
4. immobility, cigarette smoking, surgical procedures.
5. rest and sleep.
6. acetylcysteine (Mucomyst).
7. codeine, hydrocodone, hydromorphone, morphine.
8. rebound nasal congestion.

9. increase.
10. nausea, vomiting, constipation, dizziness, drowsiness, pruritus, drug dependence.
11. MAO inhibitors.
12. blow his or her nose.
13. just before feeding.
14. 30 minutes.
15. 2000–3000 ml.

**Crossword puzzle**

*Across*

3. Acetaminophen.
4. Rhinitis.
7. Acetylcysteine.
8. Antitussive.
9. Dimetapp.
10. Robitussin.

*Down*

1. Nasal.
2. Dextromethorpan.
5 Sudafed.
6. Organidin.

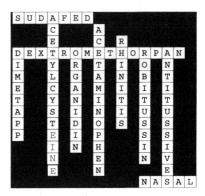

**Review questions**

1. d.
2. b.
3. c.
4. b.
5. c.
6. a.
7. b.
8. d.
9. d.
10. b.

## CHAPTER 53
### Physiology of the Cardiovascular System

**Matching exercise: terms and concepts**

1. B.
2. E.
3. G.
4. F.
5. C.
6. A.
7. K.
8. L.
9. O.
10. P.
11. Q.
12. T.
13. R.
14. S.
15. V.

**Review questions**

1. a.
2. c.
3. d.
4. c.
5. d.
6. a.
7. b.
8. d.
9. d.
10. a.

## CHAPTER 54
### Cardiotonic-Inotropic Agents Used in Congestive Heart Failure

**Complete the following sentences**

1. increases; increases; vasoconstriction. increases; increases; ventricular hypertrophy.
2. preload.
3. increase; slow.
4. fibrillation, flutter.
5. 1–1.5 mg
6. 0.1 mg.
7. 0.057 mg.
8. (Inocor); short-term.
9. cardiac arrhythmias.
10. 20–30%
11. arrhythmias.
12. digitalis effects.
13. digoxin toxicity.
14. a. arrhythmias.
    b. anorexia, nausea, vomiting.
    c. headache, drowsiness, confusion.
    d. visual disturbances.
15. a. thrombocytopenia.
    b. anorexia, nausea, vomiting.
    c. hypotension.
    d. hepatotoxicity.

**Matching exercise: terms and concepts**

1. F.
2. H.
3. K.
4. A.
5. E.
6. G.
7. M.
8. D.
9. J.
10. I.
11. L

**Review questions**

1. a.
2. b.
3. a.
4. b.
5. c.
6. d.
7. b.
8. c.
9. d.
10. c.

## CHAPTER 55
### Antiarrhythmic Drugs

**Matching exercise: terms and concepts**

1. B.
2. A.
3. F.
4. G.
5. J.
6. M.
7. L.
8. E.
9. D.
10. C.

**Crossword puzzle**

*Across*

9. Digoxin.
10. Disopyramide.

*Down*

1. Quinidine.
2. Propranolol.
3. Pronestyl.
4. Brevibloc.
5. Lidocaine.
6. Bretylium.
7. Atropine.
8. Verapamil.

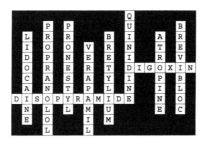

**Cardiac electrophysiology**

*Part A. Diagram completion*

1. Left atrium.
2. Left ventricle.
3. Left bundle branch.
4. Purkinje's fibers.
5. Right bundle branch.
6. Bundle of His.
7. Right ventricle.
8. A-V node.
9. Right atrium.
10. S-A node.

*Part B. Drug effect on cardiac physiology*

1. 7. Right ventricle.
2. 10. S-A node; 8. A-V node.
3. 8. A-V node; 6. Bundle of His, 5. Right bundle branch, 7. Right ventricle, 3. Left bundle branch, 2. Left ventricle.
4. 10. S-A node; 8. A-V node.

**Arrhythmia analysis exercise**

1. supraventricular tachycardia; Brevibloc.
2. atrial fibrillation; Lanoxin.
3. bradycardia; atropine.
4. premature ventricular contractions; Xylocaine.

**Review questions**

1. d.
2. b.
3. b.
4. c.
5. c.
6. c.
7. a.
8. a.
9. a.
10. c.
11. d.
12. c.

## CHAPTER 56
### Antianginal Drugs

1. Venous pressure and venous return to the heart; blood volume and blood pressure (preload); cardiac workload; oxygen demand. flow to the myocardium; peripheral resistance.
2. heart rate; myocardial contractility, blood pressure, myocardial workload, oxygen demand.
3. Coronary, peripheral arteries; myocardial contractility.
4. heavy meals, cigarette smoking, strenuous exercise.
5. diet, adequate rest.
6. 5; 3. see their physician.
7. hypotension, dizziness, headaches.
8. hypotension, bradycardia, bronchospasm, congestive heart failure.
9. a. X.
   b. X.
   c.
   d. X.
   e.
   f.
   g. X.
10. avoid strenuous exercise; assume a prone position.

**Matching exercise: terms and concepts**

1. E.
2. B.
3. G.
4. A.
5. I.
6. H.
7. K.
8. C.
9. F.
10. I.

**Review questions**

1. a.
2. d.
3. c.
4. b.
5. b.
6. a.
7. c.
8. d.
9. b.
10. c.

## CHAPTER 57
### Drugs Used in Hypotension and Shock

**True or false**

1. F.
2. F.
3. T.
4. T.
5. F.
6. T.
7. F.
8. T.
9. F.
10. T.

**Complete the following sentences**

1. decreased; decreased; decreased.
2. peripheral vascular resistance.
3. myocardial contractility, heart rate.
4. 90/60; 50 ml/hr.
5. phentolamine (Regitine).

**Review questions**

1. b.
2. c.
3. a.
4. d.
5. c.
6. b.
7. b.
8. b.
9. d.
10. b.

## CHAPTER 58
### Antihypertensive Drugs

**Match the drug group with its effect**

1. E.
2. A.
3. F.
4. B.
5. C.
6. D.
7. G.

**Match the antihypertensive medication with the group it is intended for**

1. D.
2. E.
3. A.
4. C.
5. B.

**True or false**

1. T.
2. F.
3. F.
4. T.
5. T.

**Name That Drug**

1. Captopril (Capoten).
2. Diazoxide (Hyperstat).
3. Sodium nitroprusside (Nipride).
4. Hydrochlorothiazide (Hydrodiuril).
5. Beta blockers.
6. Beta blockers, calcium channel blockers.
7. Vasodilators.
8. Clonidine (Catapres).
9. Diet and exercise.
10. Antiadrenergics, vasodilators, ACE inhibitors plus loop diuretics.
11. Thiazide diuretics.
12. Reserpine (Serpasil).
13. Clonidine (Catapres), guanabenz (Wytensin).
14. Enalapril (Vasotec), lisinopril (Zestril).
15. hydralazine (Apresoline).
16. Nonselective beta blockers, propranolol (Inderal).

**Review questions**

1. b.
2. c.
3. c.
4. d.
5. a.
6. b.
7. a.
8. a.
9. b.
10. d.

## CHAPTER 59
### Diuretics

**Complete the following sentences**

1. glomerular-filtration, tubular reabsorption, tubular secretion.
2. 400 ml; normal amounts; metabolic end products.
3. proximal tubule.
4. Antidiuretic hormone; water.
5. Aldosterone; sodium; potassium.
6. uric acid, creatinine, hydrogen ions, ammonia.
7. potassium ions, hydrogen ions, ammonia.
8. increased capillary permeability, increased capillary hydrostatic pressure, decreased plasma osmotic pressure.
9. tissue fluids; decreasing plasma volume.
10. peripheral vascular resistance; sodium; have a vasodilating effect on arterioles.
11. Thiazide diuretics; 2.
12. sodium; potassium. Hyperkalemia.
13. solute load (osmotic pressure); water; bloodstream. Mannitol.
14. electrolytes, uric acid, blood glucose, creatinine, BUN.
15. blood pressure, weight, urine output, edematous extremities.
16. digoxin toxicity; diuretic-induced hypokalemia.
17. 3.5–5.0 mEq/liter.
18. giving supplemental potassium, giving potassium-sparing diuretic, increasing [potassium] intake, salt substitutes, restricting sodium.
19. ECG changes, dysrhythmias, hypotension, weak shallow respiration, anorexia, nausea, vomiting, paralytic ileus, skeletal muscle weakness, confusion, disorientation.

**True or false**

1. F.
2. T.
3. T.
4. F.
5. F.

The nephron
1. Efferent arteriole.
2. Afferent arteriole.
3. Bowman's capsule.
4. Glomerulus.
5. Distal tubule.
6. Proximal tubule.
7. Collecting tubule.
8. Descending limb of loop of Henle.
9. Ascending limb of loop of Henle.
10. Loop of Henle.

**Review questions**

1. c.
2. a.
3. a.
4. a.
5. a.
6. b.
7. b.
8. d.
9. b.
10. c.

## CHAPTER 60
### Anticoagulant, Antiplatelet, and Thrombolytic Agents

**Complete the Chart**

**Drug:** Heparin
**Mechanism of Action:** Inactivates clotting factors IX, X, XI, XII and thrombin; prevents thrombus formation.
**Antidote:** Protamine
**Administration:** IV or SC
**Lab Test:** APPT.
**Onset of Action:** Onset immediate

**Drug:** Warfarin sodium (Coumadin)
**Mechanism of Action:** Acts on the liver to prevent the formation of vitamin-K–dependent clotting factors.
**Antidote:** Vitamin K
**Administration:** PO, rarely IM or IV
**Lab Test:** PTT.
**Onset of Action:** Onset 3–5 days

**Drug:** Aspirin
**Mechanism of Action:** Inhibits synthesis of prostaglandins; prevents formation of thromboxame $A_2$; prevents platelet aggregation.
**Antidote:**
**Administration:** PO
**Lab Test:**
**Onset of Action:**

**Drug:** Streptokinase
**Mechanism of Action:** Breaks down fibrin.
**Antidote:** Amicar
**Administration:** IV
**Lab Test:**
**Onset of Action:** Onset immmediate

**Identify whether the following drugs increase or decrease the effects of Coumadin**

1. Increase.
2. Increase.
3. Decrease.
4. Decrease.
5. Increase.
6. Decrease.
7. Increase.
8. Increase.
9. Decrease.
10. Decrease or increase.

## Review questions

1. c.
2. c.
3. c.
4. d.
5. b.
6. d.
7. d.
8. a.
9. a.
10. a.

## CHAPTER 61
### Antilipemics and Peripheral Vasodilators

**Match the drug with its side effects**

1. C.
2. B.
3. D.
4. A.
5. F.
6. E.

**True or false**

1. T.
2. T.
3. F.
4. T.
5. F.
6. T.
7. F.
8. F.
9. T.
10. T.

## Review questions

1. d.
2. a.
3. c.
4. d.
5. a.
6. b.
7. b.
8. c.
9. c.
10. a.

## CHAPTER 62
### Physiology of the Digestive System

**Matching exercise: terms and oncepts**

1. D.
2. E.
3. F.
4. G.
5. A.
6. I.
7. K.
8. B.
9. C.
10. M.
11. N.
12. O.
13. P.
14. Q.
15. R.

## Review questions

1. c.
2. b.
3. a.
4. d.
5. a.
6. d.
7. b.
8. c.
9. b.
10. a.

## CHAPTER 63
### Drugs Used in Peptic Ulcer Disease

**Matching exercise: terms and concepts**

1. B.
2. C.
3. D.
4. A.
5. E.
6. F.
7. I.
8. H.
9. G.
10. J.

**True or false**

1. T.
2. F.
3. F.
4. F.
5. F.

**Complete the following sentences**

1. reflux esophagitis, gastritis, heartburn.
2. gastric acid.
3. the amount; acidity.
4. potent; drug interactions.
5. Pepcid; Axid; mental confusion, gynecomastia.
6. Cytotec; GI bleeding.
7. Carafate; ulcer; coating; healing.
8. a. cigarette smoking.
   b. physiological stress.
   c. psychological stress.
   d. genetic influences.
   e. sex.
   f. drug therapy.

**Match the following drugs that interact with cimetidine (Tagamet) with their classification.**

1. D.
2. F.
3. C.
4. G.
5. E.
6. B.
7. H.
8. A.

**Crossword puzzle**

*Across*

7. Prostaglandins.
9. Aluminum.
10. Calcium.

*Down*

1. Omeprazole.
2. Palatability.
3. Hypersecretion.
4. Sucralfate.
5. Misoprostol.
6. Cimetidine.
8. Sodium.

## Review questions

1. a.
2. b.
3. b.
4. a.
5. d.
6. d.
7. c.
8. b.
9. a.
10. d.

## CHAPTER 64
### Laxatives and Cathartics

**Matching exercise: terms and concepts**

1. F.
2. E.
3. A.
4. D.
5. G.
6. B.
7. H.
8. C.
9. I.
10. J.
11. L.
12. N.
13. O.
14. Q.
15. P.

**Review questions**

1. a.
2. c.
3. a.
4. c.
5. c.
6. b.
7. b.
8. d.
9. c.
10. c.

## CHAPTER 65
### Antidiarrheals

**True or false**

1. F.
2. T.
3. T.
4. T.
5. F.
6. T.
7. T.
8. F.
9. T.
10. F.
11. T.
12. F.
13. F.
14. F.
15. T.

**Review questions**

1. a.
2. d.
3. a.
4. b.
5. a.
6. c.
7. d.
8. b.
9. c.
10. b.

## CHAPTER 66
### Antiemetics

**Matching exercise: terms and concepts**

1. J.
2. A.
3. I.
4. B.
5. C.
6. H.
7. D.
8. G.
9. E.
10. F.

**Review questions**

1. a.
2. d.
3. b.
4. b.
5. d.
6. c.
7. a.
8. b.
9. b.
10. a.

## CHAPTER 67
### Antineoplastics

**Matching exercise: terms and concepts**

1. D.
2. J.
3. A.
4. I.
5. B.
6. H.
7. G.
8. F.
9. C.
10. E.

11. L.
12. K.
13. O.
14. M.
15. N.

**True or false**

1. F.
2. T.
3. F.
4. T.
5. T.
6. T.
7. F.
8. T.
9. T.
10. T.
11. F.
12. T.
13. F.
14. F.
15. T.

**Review questions**

1. d.
2. b.
3. c.
4. c.
5. a.
6. b.
7. c.
8. c.
9. a.
10. d.

## CHAPTER 68
### Drugs Used in Ophthalmic Conditions

**Matching exercise: terms and concepts**

1. E.
2. D.
3. C.
4. B.
5. A.
6. J.
7. F.
8. G.
9. I.
10. H.

**Complete the following sentences**

1. anticholinergics, antihistamines, antipsychotics.
2. inflammatory conditions.
3. decreases.
4. dye.
5. Pilocarpine (Pilocar); 4; constrict.
6. dilate; glaucoma.
7. up; lower lid; conjunctival sac.
8. irritation, discomfort, lacrimation, contact dermatitis.
9. cataract formation.
10. decreased vision in dim light.

**Name that drug**

1. Osmotic diuretics.
2. Miotics.
3. Anticholinergics.
4. Carbonic anhydrase inhibitors.
5. Adrenergic mydriatrics.

**Drug classification**

1. Dipivefrin (Propine); glaucoma examinations, uveitis, pre- and post-op local hemostasis.
2. Timolol maleate (Timoptic); glaucoma.
3. Pilocarpine (Pilocar); glaucoma.
4. Physostigmine salicylate (Isopto Eserine); glaucoma.
5. Atropine sulfate; examinations, pre- and post-op uveitis, secondary glaucoma.
6. Acetazolamide (Diamox); glaucoma, pre-op.
7. Glycerin (Osmoglyn); pre-op, acute glaucoma.
8. Benoxinate hydrochloride (Dorsacaine); tonometry, removal of sutures and foreign bodies.
9. Cromolyn sodium (Opticrom); allergic keratitis, conjunctivitis.
10. Silver nitrate; prophylaxis of gonorrhea.

**Review questions**

1. a.
2. a.
3. d.
4. a.
5. c.
6. b.
7. c.
8. d.
9. c.
10. a.

## CHAPTER 69
### Drugs Used in Dermatologic Conditions

**Matching exercise: terms and concepts**

1. N.
2. A.
3. M.
4. B.
5. L.
6. C.
7. K.
8. D.
9. J.
10. E.
11. F.
12. T.
13. G.
14. H.
15. O.
16. T.
17. P.
18. S.
19. Q.
20. R.

**Review questions**

1. c.
2. b.
3. a.
4. d.
5. b.
6. a.
7. a.
8. b.
9. a.
10. d.

**CHAPTER 70**
**Drug Use During Pregnancy and Lactation**

**Place an *X* next to the drugs that should be avoided during pregnancy**

1.
2. X
3.
4. X
5. X
6.
7.
8. X
9.
10. X
11. X
12. X

**Matching exercise: terms and concepts**

1. F.
2. A.
3. E.
4. B.
5. C.
6. E.

**Complete the following sentences**

*Normal Pregnancy*

1. increases.
2. 50 [%] increase; increase.
3. anemia.
4. increase.
5. Increased.
6. Decreased
7. Increased.

*Pregnancy-Induced Hypertension*

1. edema.
2. anemia.
3. BP.
4. Decreased.
5. Increased, retention of, decreased.

**Crossword puzzle**

*Across*

3. Tocolytic.
9. Acetaminophen.
10. Insulin.

*Down*

1. Oxytocin.
2. Digoxin.
4. Lactation.
5. Bromocriptine.
6. Methyldopa.
7. Brain.
8. Meperidine.

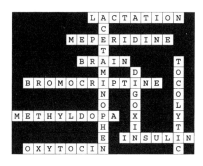

**Review questions**

1. a.
2. a.
3. b.
4. d.
5. d.
6. c.
7. b.
8. c.
9. b.
10. b.